SEXUAL INTIMACY

A guide to explore desire and sex game for couples, sexual fantasies in marriage and same-sex couples. What women and men really want from sex. Tips, massage, positions

DONNA DARE

© **Copyright 2019 - All rights reserved.**

The content contained within this book may not be reproduced, duplicated or transmitted without direct written permission from the author or the publisher.

Under no circumstances will any blame or legal responsibility be held against the publisher, or author, for any damages, reparation, or monetary loss due to the information contained within this book. Either directly or indirectly.

Legal Notice:

This book is copyright protected. This book is only for personal use. You cannot amend, distribute, sell, use, quote or paraphrase any part, or the content within this book, without the consent of the author or publisher.

Disclaimer Notice:

Please note the information contained within this document is for educational and entertainment purposes only. All effort has been executed to present accurate, up to date, and reliable, complete information. No warranties of any kind are declared or implied. Readers acknowledge that the author is not engaging in the rendering of legal, financial, medical or professional advice. The content within this book has been derived from various sources. Please consult a licensed professional before attempting any techniques outlined in this book.

By reading this document, the reader agrees that under no circumstances is the author responsible for any losses, direct or indirect, which are incurred as a result of the use of information contained within this document, including, but not limited to, — errors, omissions, or inaccuracies.

Table of Contents

Description 1

Introduction 3
    Learning to Touch 5
    The Active Role and the Liability 6
    Awakening the Sensations 7
    Be Acierated from Front and Backs 9

Chapter 1: How Communicate with Your Partner 11

Chapter 2: Developing Your Sexual Relationship with Your Partner 14

Chapter 3: Clearing the Decks for Sex 27
    Tempus fugit (time flies) 28
    Making time your bitch 29
    Back to that "roommate" thing 33

Chapter 4: Explore Him/Her Body 35
    The Female Body 35
    The Male Body 50

Chapter 5: How to Give an Erotic Massage to Help Increase Intimacy 57

Chapter 6: Unlocking Intimate Capacity Through Synergy 65

Chapter 7: Spicy And Dirty Talk 81

Chapter 8: Masturbation 90
    How to Enjoy it to the Maximum 91
    In Solitude 92
    In Couple 93

Chapter 9: Orgasms 96

Chapter 10: Sex Toys: What Choose For Him And For Her 110

Chapter 11: Using Props During Sex 121

Chapter 12: Sexual And Aphrodisiac Food 128

    Chocolate.. 128

    Horseradish... 129

    Pomegranates 132

    Bananas 133

Chapter 13: The Intricacies of Pleasure and Orgasms 135

    Stage 1 – Excitement (time frame: A few minutes to several hours) 138

    Stage 2 – Plateau 139

    Stage 3 – Orgasm... 140

    Stage 4 – Resolution 141

Chapter 14: The Most Intimate Positions For Couple 144

Conclusion... 164

Description

Finding time to spice things up in a relationship can be difficult and it takes work. If you want to keep things fun and sexy then you must put in the work. Trying new positions and incorporating new sex toys will keep things hot and heavy between you and your partner. Learning about each other and finding what feels good and what turns each other on is crucial. Taking a trip to a local sex shop or surfing the net for new sex positions is a great way to eliminate the boring sex life that you may have and create a better sexual experience for the two of you. Try new things! This may be intimidating at first but once you become more comfortable with each other it will be much easier.

The fun in having sex involves getting to know each other, your bodies and what feels good for the other person. When you are able to provide your partner with an immense amount of pleasure, this feeling alone is a turn on. Watch the facial expressions of your partner as you lift them up, bend them over, and straddle them or whatever else you do to make them feel good. Allow this moment to turn you on. Most of all, have fun! Sex is a sensual moment for two individuals, but it's also a great way to release stress and feel good. When you have an orgasm, you release tension. Let go of daily stress by making it a point to have sex a few times a week. Make time for this! Great sexual relationships take time and commitment to the task at hand. The task of providing pleasure for another individual is a great thing, but it's also an experience that will open new doors for new ways of receiving pleasure and fulfillment from your partner.

This guide will focus on the following:

- How to communicate with your partner
- Developing your sexual relationship with your partner
- Clearing the decks for sex
- Explore him/her body
- How to give an erotic massage to help increase intimacy
- Unlocking intimate capacity through synergy
- Spicy and dirty talk
- Masturbation
- Orgasms
- Sex toys: what choose for him and for her
- Using props during sex
- Sexual and aphrodisiac food
- The intricacies of pleasure and orgasms
- The most intimate positions for couples... AND MORE!!!

Introduction

A good lover is one who is willing to give her pleasure and who enjoys feeling how desire grows in her. He is attentive to her reactions, without assuming that what has made her or another woman enjoy before is a kind of universal recipe that will always be exciting. In general, it is the one who is sensitive to know how you want to be stimulated, in particular.

Although there are clear responses of desire with direct contact in the erotic points, female psychology can be governed by rejection when the caresses are mechanical, or if they perceive the lover's hurry to erotize them and accelerate the moment of penetration. It leads her to think that he only wishes to stimulate them in search of his own pleasure.

Being more flexible than men, they launch themselves into new games and fantasies, so when they are the ones that are stimulating them, they quickly learn to satisfy them; but they expect and need him to do the same. The ideal lover is the one who is able to notice the subtle changes in the feminine mood. There are women who carefully choose underwear as a claim of seduction and get frustrated if he only notices but doesn't comment. The woman has a more developed feeling of erotic correspondence, so she knows that pleasure does not depend on the sensual capacity of one of the lovers, but on both.

What makes her sexual desires grow more is that as her desire and arousal increase, he should make her feel special and desired. For her, the small details are as important as the big gestures in any sexual encounter. Their morbidness wakes up to situations that escape the routine as when they are caressed while still dressed or half-undressed. Situations that are set aside from the bedroom, moments that remind them of their first sexual scuffles or when lovers run the risk of being surprised. Their fantasies are also triggered if the caresses are not predictable and mechanical friction in the breasts or vulva are avoided. This sensitive mode of the approach causes her to intensely see the stimulation of the erogenous points and begin to crave contact.

One of the attitudes that the woman values and that makes her sexual cravings grow is that, as her desire and excitement increases, he makes her feel that she also enjoys, prolonging the stimulus for her to enjoy.

In certain men, impatience is noticeable or they seem to get bored if the woman is slow to get excited, acting as if they were spectators waiting for penetration to begin. This can cause the woman's libido to retract.

However, the most important thing a good lover should know is that the woman is different in her sexuality, more complex and much more subtle. A direct stimulus in the erogenous zones and the enjoyment he obtains through penetration is enough for him since his sexuality is more direct. It is easy for him to reach an allegory. She needs, instead, the mystery and the display of imagination because she does not care about the number of orgasms, or sexual athletics, but the degree of eroticism.

Learning to Touch

Touching the lover for the simple pleasure of doing so, feeling his reaction and perceiving the touch of firmer, elastic or tender skin, awakens perceptions that move, disturb, or excite. But above all, touching is the intense enjoyment of knowing each other without having the precise objective of intercourse or orgasm.

The big secret is to turn the touches into a purpose in themselves. Turn it into a creative game, free and without rules, in which everything goes. There are no allowed or prohibited areas. The flexibility and disinhibition that this seeks are difficult to equate to any other form of knowledge. It is the purest enjoyment that pleases the sensitivity and the exciting territory of the skin.

The Active Role and the Liability

The pleasure of being touched is not less than that which is felt by caressing the lover. Therefore, the ductile and natural exchange of roles brings a playful aspect to eroticism. It is intensely sensual to assume an active attitude seeking to stimulate the other, who gives himself to the pleasure of caress enjoying the situation joyfully. Likewise, the inverse attitude is equally exciting. In this way, not being aware or being routine in the role that is assumed allows each encounter between lovers to contain a subliminal expectation.

She intertwines her arms around his neck or waist, supports her hips while standing and facing each other, playing an active role and conveying her need to feel him very close, as well as being tightly embraced, trapped, and protected. Although the active role is usually identified with masculinity, the truth is that this depends on the psychological profile of each person, whether man or woman.

Self-Carry

The woman, no matter how liberated, finds it difficult to stop associating the caresses in her own body with masturbation. He also has a hard time doing it in front of his lover. Stroking for pure pleasure is the first step to discover new sensations and in every inch of your body.

In the beginning, the caresses should be soft and slow. The arms or legs are a good starting point. The skin will respond to the touches expressing, in its own way, when it needs the rhythm or intensity to vary. Then different types of friction are experienced and alternated: with the open hand, with the fingertips, with greater depth, as if there were small taps, with the knuckles, the back of the hands, with the nails or running with tissues of various textures such as feathers, velvets, and silks.

Awakening the Sensations

Once the game of caresses begins, they become combined, form a chain, and respond to the rhythm that flows freely. He is going to touch the breasts or the back, but he grazes the neck by chance and that changes the planned route. He hears a murmur of pleasure that ignites her and feels the promise of enjoyment offered by that point to his hands, his lips, and his tongue. To her, that exciting contact encourages her to respond by stroking his body or shaking it to feel it closer.

He kisses her softly and affectionately. He only wants to comfort her but she incites him by kissing him, biting, and sucking his mouth. Once the instinct is triggered, it does not resist and descends through the excited body to more vulnerable points that await its touches with deep anxiety.

Imagination is a good ally to transmit caresses to certain unusual body parts, which is sensual contact, offer unknown pleasures. Feel the firmness of a knee stroking the soft inside of the thighs, the nipples sliding down the belly or the female back, the hand that, without stroking, encloses the pubis and the entire vulva in a tight and warm wrap intimate, are some suggestions which will help you to not fall into repetition. The true awakening achieved by touching is one of the plateaus of enjoyment, a point in the path of pleasure.

Be Acierated from Front and Backs

Sometimes, caresses begin with clothes out of which, little by little, one strips off. The nakedness communicates between the skin of one and the other a contact which is not only sensual but also of a great emotionality. Some parts of the female body are largely forgotten, usually because of the positions that are adopted. It is the case of the back that, due to the multiple nerve endings that run through the center and along the spine, when touched, responds vividly. She is lying on her stomach and her back is in view; he caresses her with alternating touches. Worrying about aesthetic perfection often limits the pleasure you feel, given the possibility of feeling rejection from it. Actually, a man does not give much importance to this issue, but his sexuality awakens first and that sets some unsaid parameters. Imagination is a good ally to transmit caresses to certain unusual body parts.

The most exciting sensations wake up when a caress or casual touch finds an exact point of sensitivity that remained hidden and that, once stimulated, provides a surprise and unexpected pleasure. He caresses those with the hands, then rubs it with the knuckles, inserts taps, kisses, and licks between the shoulder blades, in the center, until reaching the edge of the waist, without advancing in principle beyond. She moves sensually, feels relaxed, and stimulated at the same time.

He continues to play downstream, palpate the buttocks, and traces its contour with an unprinted finger to caress with passion. It is as if he is drawing its shape. He then reaches the legs, passes the fingertips lightly through the soft inside of the thighs, and reaches the calves, caresses them, and then takes the sensitive toes one by one and kisses them warmly. If she seems pleased and he notices her relaxed body, he gently incorporates it until she is seated. Then, standing behind her, he caresses her breasts, initiating the soft and very slow touch at first without directly looking for the nipples. Their movements are enveloping and rotating. You can also simply hold the breasts between the palms of the hands.

After a prolonged and intense caressing session of him, she wishes to participate by caressing herself or returning the caresses. If self-stimulation is reduced to a simple sexual discharge alone, sexuality is impoverished.

Chapter 1: How Communicate with Your Partner

It is true. Communication is the key to any successful relationship. Especially when it comes to something like Kamasutra. It is the duty of each partner to ensure that they are satisfying their lover, but it is also their duty to let their lover know how they are feeling.

Humans are not minded readers, and often times do not know what you are thinking. You have to be open with your partner and allow your partner to be open with you. Otherwise, you will have some serious issues. A lot of times people are not open because their partners shut them down, and get angry at criticism, so they feel that they are not able to be open. You have to encourage communication both in and out of the bedroom.

In the bedroom, make your partner feel comfortable with vocalization. If they are nervous, let them know that it is not silly, and you like knowing that what you are doing feels good, or if it doesn't feel good, you want to know so that you can make the proper adjustments. You should also lead by example. A lot of times one partner is very vocal, while the other is silent, you should both be vocal. Do not be afraid of shouting or screaming in pleasure. Also, do not be scared to tell your partner what doesn't feel good. You can make it less harsh by asking them to change something nicely, rather than saying that hurts. This way there is no killing of the mood.

You also need communication in your everyday life as well. When your partner upsets you, you should tell them rather than bottling it up until it becomes a fight. You should also tell them if they are doing something you like. Too many times in the real world, everyone talks about what they don't like, but no one talks about what they do like. Yet in the bedroom, it is the opposite. You should definitely find a balance in both.

Communication is a necessary part of your everyday life. Even if it is just talking about your day. Many relationships fail because there is not enough communication to keep the passion alive. You want to tell your partner everything. When they ask how your day was, it is because they want to know. They do not want a one-word answer such as "good." When they ask you, be free with the information. Tell them every little boring detail, and then ask them about their day.

Revel in what they are saying to you, even if the words are unimportant. Your lover will be happy knowing that even if they had a really boring day, you want to know about it. Things like that are the little things that make the world go round, and indeed make a relationship work. Communication is a show of love, and it will help keep your love strong. Use it to its fullest power.

Chapter 2: Developing Your Sexual Relationship with Your Partner

It can be intimidating making that transition from simply flirting into a full-blown sexual relationship with your partner, but it is good to know that for most couples, the more sex that they have the better the relationship becomes when it is based on mutual respect trust and love. Before having sex with anyone, it is important that you are completely comfortable discussing sexual affairs with that person and that you are 100% ready for that step. Do not allow yourself to be pressured into making any decisions because the only right time to move to that stage in your relationship is when both people are on the same page about sexual intimacy.

When Is the Best Time to Have Sex for the First Time?

This is a complicated question, and the right answer varies from person to person and relationship to relationship. To some people, the answer is the very first day that they meet someone. To others, that right answer maybe a few weeks or months into dating someone. Not before marriage is the right answer to other people. While the answer to this is complicated, one thing for sure is that sex should not be engaged in unless both parties are completely ready for the act. This is especially true if you are a virgin and have never had sex before.

Tips for Having Sex with Your Partner for the First Time

The initial stages of exploring your sexual attraction to your partner can be filled with excitement and adventure as you learn what each other's turn-on are, explore each other's bodies, and tap into each other's sexual fantasies. However, before you just dive in, be sure to have a discussion about sexual boundaries, meaning what you both are okay with engaging in the bedroom. Both of you need to be frank and open about what works for you sexually and what does not. By eliminating the worry that your partner might unknowingly go into territory that you are not comfortable with, you can both simply enjoy the moment and being together.

The first time that sexual penetration occurs in a relationship can be particularly anxiety-provoking for some couples. It may be the first time that you completely bare your body and, therefore, your vulnerabilities and insecurities to that person. However, no matter how intimidating that moment may be, it should be something that is supremely enjoyable for both you and your partner. To ensure that this is the case, I have compiled a few tips to ensure that your first time goes as smoothly as possible.

- *Get into a relaxed state of mind before the date.* While the first time can be a spontaneous event, most couples know exactly when the first time will be. Being tense will make this an awkward and probably unfulfilling event. Therefore, prepare yourself mentally with simple meditation or yoga techniques to soothe any nerves that you might have. Think of it as a pre-sex warm-up.

- *Wear clothing and underwear that makes you feel sexy.* Knowing that you look good will feed your self-confidence at the moment. This does not automatically mean that you should wear thong underwear or exaggerated lingerie pieces. Sexual attractiveness and comfort should go hand-in-hand. Make sure that you look good *and* feel good in what you are wearing.

- *Do not focus on your appearance.* Sometimes we focus too much on how we appear during the active sexual intercourse such as wondering if a position flatters us or if the lighting compliments us, and we don't focus enough on how we feel at that moment. Remember that your partner is with you at that moment because he or she is already attracted to you. Just focus on your enjoyment of the moment.

- *Take your time and make-out first.* Anxiety and pure horniness can make you feel like you need to rush to the main event for the first time but resist the temptation and allow the tension to build with a pre-sex make-out session. Since this is your first time with your partner, make it something that you will remember forever. Savor each sensation and every moment. By taking your time and making the moment last for as long as possible, you both get as aroused as possible and are both more likely to orgasm from the session.

- *Bring protection.* Do not just leave it up to your partner to take on the responsibility of ensuring that you have protection. You are both equally responsible, and if that person happens to not have any, you can be assured that you have got things covered.

- *Do not be afraid to voice your needs and ask questions.* If your partner is doing something that you really like, do not be afraid to tell them so. The same goes for if they are doing something that you do not like. Instead of being worried about if your actions are pleasing to them, simply speak up and ask. It is important to build your sexual communication skills right off the bat in any relationship, and it is no different for your first time.

- *Laughter is good.* Sometimes sex can be funny. Maybe it is an awkward position, bumping your foreheads together, or the dreaded queef that arouses a moment of hilarity. Whatever it may be, do not be afraid to laugh. Not only does this beat awkward and not put too much pressure on the moment but it also helps bring you two closer.

- *Do not bring up past lovers or past sexual encounters.* I think this goes without saying but most people do not like being compared to someone's past sexual partners even if the comparison is done to show that they are better. By doing this you will only make the moment weird, so do not do it.

- *Do not focus on your orgasm.* This is especially useful advice for women. This is not to say that orgasming is not important; however, putting too much pressure on reaching it can be the reason why it does not happen. Do not focus on the big finish but rather on enjoying yourself at the moment.

Masturbation for Couples

Another first that many couples encounter in their sexual relationship is shared masturbation. Before we get into how masturbation can improve your relationships, let's tackle a few myths about the act. It is simply not true that masturbation will:

- Cause you to go blind or make your eyesight go bad.
- Cause the male penis to shrink in size.
- Make you go insane.
- Cause cancer.
- Give you an STD.
- Cause you to become homosexual or adopt a homosexual lifestyle.

- Hinder your social and emotional development.
- Make you sterile.
- Make you unfaithful.

I do admit that some of these myths border on ridiculous; however, many people do believe in them, and it is important that we educate as many people on sexual topics. It is true that masturbation can be harmful to a relationship if it is done in the wrong way. You will know that you are doing it wrong if:

- You have to hide the fact that you do engage in masturbation from your partner.
- You look forward to masturbation more than you look forward to being sexually active with your partner.
- You substitute masturbation for intimacy with your partner.
- You masturbate to the point of self-injury.
- Masturbation interferes with your personal and work life.
- You feel shame regarding the act because of religious beliefs, family views, or media messages.

- You have tried to stop masturbating at such a high frequency and have been unsuccessful at stopping or decreasing the amount of time that you spend doing it.

In such cases, while masturbation can indeed affect your relationship, this is an issue that needs to be dealt with individually. It is a great idea to seek the help of a therapist and enlist the help of your partner so that you can get the help you need.

The negative outcomes of masturbation on a relationship can include the promotion of feelings of inadequacy. This is a consequence when one partner hides that they engage in masturbation and the other party finds out. The person who finds out may feel that their partner is bored or unhappy with them as a sexual partner, and this may give rise to insecurities. It can also give rise to distrust. If indeed one party was engaging in masturbation in secret, the other party may feel that they cannot trust this person because they have kept such an important aspect about themselves secret.

As you can see from all of the negative incomes above, masturbation that is done in secret and without communication with the other party is detrimental to a relationship. By being open and honest about your needs and exploring the satisfaction that masturbation can bring, you can open the door for an even healthier, more active sex life with your partner. Again, it all starts with effective communication.

Getting the courage to masturbate in front of your partner can also be intimidating because of body issues and revealing so much of yourself to someone but masturbating together, which is also called mutual masturbation, can allow both of you to bare it all physically, emotionally and mentally at the same time.

Benefits of Mutual Masturbation

- You can sate your need for sexual satisfaction before you are ready to be completely intimate.

- It is a great stress reliever in long-distance relationships.

- It allows you to be sexual even if you cannot engage in penetrative sex for reasons such as risky pregnancy, risk of STD infection, or disability.

- It allows you to spice up your sex life by trying something new with your partner.

How to Masturbate Together

The first thing to do is to get comfortable. Find locations and positions that allow you to have eye contact. A particularly receptive position is to have the woman straddling the man's body. This gives both parties a full-frontal view of what is going on with the other as they masturbate at the same time. In addition to allowing each party to touch themselves, this position is great for simple touches to each other's face and chest. It also allows kissing which can increase the feeling of closeness and deepen the connection at the moment. There is also nothing wrong with giving each other a hand. The man can offer clitoral and G-spot stimulation while the woman strokes his erect penis and testicles.

There is no right way or wrong way to proceed with mutual masturbation. Do whatever feels right and good to you and your partner. If you are looking for a few ways to spice things up, here are a few ideas:

- *Add sex toys to your mutual masturbation fun.* Common sex toys include vibrators and dildos, but sex toys are not only limited to being used on women. Some men find that they like the sensation of vibrators against the skin. There is even a special sex toy for men called a stroker which fits into the hand and goes over the penis and acts as an artificial vagina. When using sex toys, be sure to use plenty of lubrication to avoid uncomfortable friction. Water-based lubricants are normally compatible with all sex toy materials.

- *Talk dirty to each other.* Dirty talk does not have to be complicated. Simply telling your partner what you are doing and how good what that person is doing feels increases the sensuality of the moment. Adding instructions can also add a dynamic of power play that some couples find very stimulating. Adding talk of fantasy is also considered dirty talk.

- *Try phone sex or do it over webcam.* This is a particularly useful tip if you are separated from your lover. Long-distance does not have to keep you from enjoying each other, and mutual masturbation is a great way to keep the sexual tension alive and well between the two of you.

- *Watch porn together and masturbate.* Many people find that watching certain porn videos arouses them, so why not use the on-screen stimulation to masturbate together? Reading erotica out loud to each other is a great alternative to this.

Oral Sex Techniques

Now that we have gotten comfortable discussing masturbation and using our hands to please each other, let's take a look at how we can use our mouths for mutual satisfaction as well. Oral sex is a beautiful expression of desire and love and can be one of the best ways for increasing sexual intimacy with your partner. This section is dedicated to helping you increase your oral sex skills to drive your partner crazy with lust and desire.

There are some general rules that apply no matter who is on the receiving end of oral sex, and they are:

- *Educate yourself.* Before you engage in oral sex, you need to be familiar with the names and functions of common sex organs such as the clitoris and the perineum. Oral sex will be a whole lot easier and more enjoyable for both parties if you eliminate ignorance.

- *Be clean as a common courtesy to your partner.* Ensure that your body and mouth are thoroughly cleaned as well as keeping facial hair and pubic hair trimmed and neat to avoid abrasion.

- *Keep bedside essentials handy.* Oral sex can be a messy affair, so it is a good practice to keep clean up devices such as tissues or wipes handy. Other items such as lubricant, hair ties for keeping long hair out of the way, sex toys, and a glass of water for the inevitable dry mouth or dehydration should be kept close as well.
- *Remember to reciprocate.* Both parties should be able to enjoy receiving oral sex, so remember to reciprocate the pleasure that your partner gives to you and vice versa.

Chapter 3: Clearing the Decks for Sex

Sex isn't something you should just "count on". That's one thing my love and I have learned over the years. For us, the initial fire hasn't so much gone out as it had to be domesticated and kept in its proper place. To be truthful, that's because we entered into our relationship with a strong awareness of how tenuous love can be. We were both committed to maintaining the quality of our bond and that meant a frank and open discussion about our sex life together, once the initial madness of love had subsided.

You know what it's like. You can't keep your hands off each other. You can barely be in the same room together, without "going there". People yell "Get a room!" at you in the street, because you're always smooching (and proudly so). Exhibitionism and day and night eroticism fuel the early bonding of all couples. Keeping that feeling alive, though, when life interrupts your mutual sexual reverie, can be a demanding and serious undertaking.

Tempus fugit (time flies)

It's no secret that the fast-paced nature of life can get in the way of our sex lives. This is especially true if you have children (babies and very young children, especially). The demands of child-rearing present their own challenges. But that's not really the focus of this book. Let's focus on ways and means of making sure you're not putting your sexuality on the back burner out of sheer laziness, cavalier neglect, or just exhaustion.

Sex in a long-term partnership can dwindle in many ways and being aware of that effect is one of the most important steps you and your partner can take to stop it from happening. The first defense against heterosexual bed death is honesty. Being honest with your partner when you sense you're neglecting each other's physical desires is key. Getting offended is a bad sign. It means you're not fully engaged and that your ego is more important to you than the health of your relationship.

Another is not making time, but taking it. Grab time by the face and make it your bitch! It's your time. It doesn't rule you. You rule it. Stop saying you don't have time. You do. You just need to move the furniture around a little to make space for sex. Sure, it's work, but any marriage/partnership requires some of that. Those who don't think that's true are probably best suited to "confirmed singledom". If you're not willing to admit that your relationship has been forged between two fallible humans, you probably should go it alone. Denying that your sex life is waning, being egotistical about approaches from your partner to address it, or laziness about doing the work involved, are not going to help. These attitudes are going to lead to the revolving door.

I'm speaking from experience. That experience, while not the most fun part of my life with my beloved, has been formative and has made me a better partner, overall and certainly, a better sex partner. So how did that experience inform us both? How did we put a stop to protestations of there never being "enough time for sex", or of being "too tired"? Most importantly, how did we do it without blaming each other, or being hurtful? Here's what we did.

Making time your bitch

My love and I are both hardworking people. One important decision we have made in our lives was not to have children. That's not for everyone. I know. But it's a decision neither of us has ever regretted, so that factor has never been a question. But work and its demands, social obligations, family and all the myriad things in life that keep us busy can build up, exhaust people and push sex to the bottom of the list. It happened to us, about four years after we began co-habiting. That's not bad, as it's a generally accepted reality that most couples experience a diminishment in sexual intensity after the first two years together.

That's right. Only two years. So if any of our relationships are to last more than two years, it's highly advisable that you take what I'm going to tell you next seriously.

At about the four-year mark, both my partner and I had continued with our careers, working hard as the General Manager of a large chain store (me) and the proprietor of a marketing consultancy (her). We were doing well, economically. We were prospering. But it was clear that focusing on our respective career paths had taken its toll. We were both tired. But more than just tired, we'd become so comfortable in each other's presence that weren't being as sensitive to one another as we'd been in the earliest layer of our relationship.

"I miss you," she said one day, over a hurried breakfast. We'd started to make a point of rising a little earlier in order to enjoy some time together in the early morning, regardless of how little of it there was.

"Me too," I replied, wistfully. We knew right then that we needed to act. My partner's tentative approach didn't lay blame. It didn't accuse. It was a simple statement of fact that got my attention. After about eight months of slow drift, with the television set numbing us into complacency, she had realized that someone needed to say something. One of us was always falling asleep in front of it – in our holey sweatpants, of course. Whoever remained awake would rouse the other before crawling off to bed – to sleep. We'd been using fatigue as an excuse to avoid the question of physical intimacy. But what was really in the way was the pacifying soporific effect of the TV.

So we turned it off for good. We loaded that sucker into the back of our SUV and drove it to the nearest Sally Ann. It was one of the best things we ever did for ourselves. Maybe some of you don't want to hear this, but that box is sucking the sexuality right out of your relationship. The time you spend staring at that thing is better spent with your partner. Some of that time is sex time. Interested now? I thought you might be.

Neilson, the company that monitors television viewing habits and derives ratings from them, conducted a study in 2014. This study revealed that the average American between the ages of 25 and 34 watches 27 and one-half hours of television, each and every week. That's more than one *day*. But if you find that figure shocking, consider this – it goes up as we age. By the time we reach the 35 – 44 brackets, we're in for 33 hours and 40 minutes. After 45, the figure rises again to almost 44 hours per week.

That is one helluva lot of time. Some couples even watch television in different rooms, exacerbating the damaging effect this modern habit can have by adding physical isolation.

I'm going to assume that most of you are in the median group (35 – 44). Can we agree that you're still young and healthy (for the most part) and sexually robust? Can we agree you're still interested in regular sex with your partner, because you're reading this book? Then maybe it's time to kick your sex-undermining little friend out of the house, for good. We did it and we're glad. We spend our time on other things, now, including sex. Sex isn't just for Saturday night at our house (although it's part of the weekend fun). Because we have exiled the insidious influence of television from our home, we are healthier, more engaged with each and happier, all around. We have time, because we've made it our bitch by making one simple change in our lives.

Back to that "roommate" thing

OK. I know sweatpants are comfortable. The thing is that if they become your home uniform, then you have effectively "de-sexified" yourself. This is true whether you are a man or a woman. Throw those things away. I mean it. My love became a bit too attached to her pair of well-worn sweats. I got to the point at which I wondered if she had lost all her other clothes, except those she wore to work. So I asked her:

"Did something happen to your other clothes?"

"No," she answered, regarding me with wide, curious eyes. "Why are you asking me that?"

As gently as possible, I asked her where the silk lounging pajamas I'd brought her from the last convention I'd attended. I told her how sexy I thought she'd look in them and asked why she never wore them.

"Those are for special occasions, honey!" She giggled, coyly.

"Every day is a special occasion, where you're concerned." I said, smiling sweetly.

Without telling her she looked like a homeless person, or dumpy, I made it clear that the sweatpants were not doing it for me; that I wanted to enjoy her glory swaddled in something perhaps more enticing than those frigging sweats. I had planned for the occasion, thought about what I intended to say and how I intended to say it, beforehand. I'd also tidied up my own appearance, in preparation. Sauce. Goose. Gander. Women are visual, too, fellas. They like to see the man they originally fell in love with, occasionally.

Chapter 4: Explore Him/Her Body

The Female Body

Many women are faced with societal pressures and social conditioning that can easily prevent them from connecting their sexual energy and engaging in sexual acts and behaviors solely for the purpose of fulfilling their own desires, rather than as an obligation to fulfill those of their partners. When a woman begins to understand that her sexuality and sexual nature are beautiful, powerful and positive, she can enjoy being sexually stimulated and nurtured by her lover. Helping her to realize her own orgasmic capacity and also be able to expand it, is one of the goals and outcomes of Tantric sex, and this chapter will explore Tantric methods and practices by which women can both be pleased by their partners.

The Yoni (Vagina)

"Yoni" (pronounced YO-nee) is the Sanskrit word for the vagina. The vagina is sacred in Tantra, and thus must be treated with the utmost care and respect. The Yoni massage is a sensuous technique that both emotionally and spiritually brings partners closer together, building trust and intimacy along the way.

How to Give a Tantric Yoni Massage

While the Yoni massage is definitely stimulating, remember that the main purpose is to relax both partners and encourage emotions to rise to the surface. Women may experience a variety of sensations and feelings during this massage ranging from lust to anger, to excitement, or indifference and all of this is a good thing! Remember, during the Yoni massage, there are no boundaries, as there is no focus on achieving any desired outcome other than to feel, observe, connect, and experience. As your skills improve and you move toward mastery of the Yoni massage, your understanding of female sexuality will deepen and your sex life as a whole will be much improved.

Breathing is a Tantric foreplay activity that assists in building emotional and spiritual bonds between lovers. Prior to beginning the Yoni massage, first spend some time increasing awareness of each other's' essence and presence by gazing into each other's eyes, embracing, and engaging in deep, synchronized breathing. The giver of the upcoming massage should take the lead in the breathing exercise, but both the giver and receiver should remain focused and relaxed during the entire activity. Should the receiver begin to stop, pause or take more shallow breaths, the giver should gently remind her of the pace and depth that she should be striving to meet.

When both parties feel sufficiently relaxed, comfortable and connected, the receiver should lie on her back with a pillow beneath her neck for comfort, and another underneath her hips, elevating her pelvis. She pulls her legs up by bending her knees with her feet flat on the bed or floor, and opens her legs, exposing her Yoni, while the giver sits cross-legged in between her open legs, on a pillow or cushion if desired.

The giver should begin by massaging other parts of her body, encouraging relaxation. Firmly and gently massage her arms, breasts, stomach, hips, and thighs before moving inward to her pelvic region. Continue by massaging her pubic bone, working your way to the inner thigh. Repeat this action, at least nine times, then use the right hand to apply a lubricant or oil to the top or mound of the Yoni, making sure that enough is poured so that the outer lips and outside of the Yoni are covered.

Rub the lubricant on the outer lips several times, as she will find this highly erotic and pleasurable. With the thumb and index finger of each hand, apply light pressure and squeeze each of her Yoni lips, sliding your oiled fingers up and down the entire length of each one. Once the outer lips are complete, repeat the process with each inner lip, paying close attention to her preferences, altering the pressure and speed according to her physical and audible cues.

The next step, clitoral stimulation, is optional and may or may not be possible, depending on her level of sensitivity to clitoral stimulation. You will have to pay close attention to her cues and expressed desires before going too far into clitoral stimulation, but if this is something that she enjoys, begin by stroking her clitoris in a gentle, circular motion. Next, while squeezing her clitoris between your thumb and index finger, rotate your hand until your wrist faces upward, carefully and slowly insert your middle finger into her Yoni, and explore the inside of her with your finger. Take your time and enjoy the way she feels. With varying degrees of speed and depth, feel up, down, right and left until you reach her "sacred spot" -- her G-spot.

Continue with the massage switching up the intensity, speed and direction. Maintain the connectivity of deep breathing and looking into each other's' eyes. At this point, she may experience waves of powerful emotion, begin to shiver, shake and cry, but no matter what, keep breathing, keep encouraging her to breathe, and remain gentle. If she does reach orgasm, ask her if she would like you to continue. At this point, if you continue, she will likely have multiple orgasms in a row, each more intense than the last. In Tantra, this exciting experience is known as "riding the wave", and many women -- even those who have never experienced orgasm before -- can learn to become multi-orgasmic when the Tantric Yoni Massage is correctly performed by a gentle, patient partner.

Your job is to keep massaging and enjoying the moment until she assures you that she is ready to stop. At that time, allow her to relish the moment and enjoy the afterglow of the powerful orgasms you have given her while you enjoy the satisfaction of pleasing your woman and creating a special moment together.

The Clitoris

The clitoris is positioned in between the labia above the vagina. It consists of two parts -- the rounded glans and the longer shaft -- which is covered by a "hood" of skin, the clitoral hood. While most, if not all, women can reach orgasm from clitoral stimulation, as stated earlier in this book, some women are too sensitive in this area so it is always a good idea to check with the woman to see how much clitoral stimulation works for her. Regardless, it is important to make sure that you use enough lubrication when venturing to manipulate any woman's clitoris. You'll never want to touch that extremely sensitive area without adequate lubrication.

How to Give a Tantric Clitoral Massage

The purpose of the Tantric clitoral massage is to make the woman's clitoris the center of attention. This massage can be given alone, as part of a Yoni massage, part of the G-spot massage (which will be covered in the next section), or part of a standard erotic massage.

If the Tantric clitoral massage is not an extension of another session where you have already set the mood, make sure to create a warming, inviting, special ambiance where your partner will feel relaxed and open. Either ask her to undress, or slowly undress her yourself, and request that she lie face down once she is fully nude. Give her a full body massage, starting on her back working your way from neck to toe. After several minutes, turn her over, and then work your back up from her feet to her shoulders and neck.

Avoid massaging her breasts or genitalia for the time being to tease her and build momentum. The goal here is to heighten her senses, keep her guessing, and to invite her to expect the unexpected.

After you have massaged every inch of her body except for her genitalia and are ready to begin the clitoral massage, gently touch either of her knees, sliding your hand up her inner thigh, continuing up to her vulva. Depending on the size and sensitivity of her clitoris, you will be massaging it using between one and three fingers. As a rule:

> a. If you can feel her clitoral shaft with your fingers, use your thumb and index finger (2 fingers).
>
> b. If her clitoris is larger and more prominent, you can use your thumb, index finger, and middle finger (3 fingers).
>
> c. On the contrary, if her clitoris is small and hidden, use either the tip of your index finger or your thumb (1 finger).

If you are only using one finger, place either the tip of your finger or your thumb atop her clitoris, move the skin underneath your finger either around in tiny circles or back and forth. Even if her clitoris is small and hidden, you should be able to feel it hardening and becoming more erect as she becomes more aroused.

If you are using more than one finger, lightly grasp the shaft with your thumb and index finger while gently sliding the tissue surrounding her clitoris back and forth in order to determine clitoral shape and firmness. It is important to determine how much the tissue around her clitoris slides around because you do not want to apply too much pressure. You want to avoid grasping the glans directly if possible, but the goal here is for the hood to slide back and forth as you manipulate the shaft, which will indirectly stimulate her glans.

Place your thumb and forefinger around the hood, lightly pinch the clitoris and gently roll it around between your fingers. Pull the hood up so that the clitoris is exposed, and blow on it. Use a heavily lubricated fingertip to gently tease it in different directions -- up, down, left, right, or in circles -- and pay attention to what she responds to best. This action will bring blood to the surface and charge her nerve endings.

If she is enjoying herself, continue in a steady rhythm. As her level of arousal increases, you can experiment with increasing pressure, but always remember to be gentle. You can vary the speed of your strokes from very slow and methodic in the beginning, making them increasingly faster as she nears orgasm.

Once she reaches orgasm, move your fingers away from her clitoris and to her labia. Maintain physical contact as she recovers from her orgasmic high. Once she has recovered you can either start over again or stop, but please never stop the massage abruptly unless she expresses discomfort. In this case, shift your focus to her vulva or other less sensitive areas in her pelvic region for a few minutes until she is ready to proceed.

Although she may orgasm very quickly and easily, it may take some time for both of you to get comfortable with this technique. The best way to figure out how to give and receive the Tantric clitoral massage is through keeping open minds and gaining experience through practicing together, which can be a great bonding experience.

The Breasts: How to Give a Tantric Breast Massage

The Tantric breast massage is a special ritual that allows a woman to receive sensual energy from her partner. Massaging the breasts makes them firmer and healthier while maintaining the hormonal balance within a woman's body. The Tantric breast massage is a way for one to please, heal and become more intimate with their partner, as the breasts need to be loved and honored first before other elements of her body will become free to open.

Breast tissue is delicate, but with proper technique and moderate pressure, a Tantric breast massage can be simple and safe. Make sure that the woman is in a warm, safe space before beginning, and verbally communicate to her that the massage is purely for her enjoyment and that she need not wonder about giving you pleasure at all.

Before beginning the massage, place one hand on her heart and the other on her Yoni and visualize energy moving from your heart into your hands and toward her heart and Yoni. This visualization is connection and healing and an important part of this Tantric massage session.

To avoid friction, apply massage oil onto the breast in circular motions going from the center of the chest into the underarm region. Caress her breasts slowly and gently, brushing the palms of your hands over the entire breast. Get into a rhythm, repeat your moves, at least twenty times at a consistent pace and pressure. First, try going clockwise on both breasts. Then try the following move:

1. Place your palm over her entire breast with the nipple in the center.

2. Fan your fingers out, mimicking a wheel spoke.

3. Slowly bring your fingers in toward the nipple.

4. Finish with a slight (or firmer if you so desire) pinch.

5. Repeat.

After the above technique is applied, the second step is to gently knead the fully covered breasts by lifting them from the chest, pressing delicately. Alternating breasts one after the other, methodically twist and wring each one in rhythmic fashion, at least twenty times.

The third step is to gently attempt to "scoop" the flesh with the flat of the fingertips; first clockwise, then counterclockwise.

Fourth, you will directly massage the nipples. Place both thumbs on opposite sides of the nipple of one breast, starting at the outside edge of her areola (the dark, flat circle surrounding her actual nipple). Slowly bring your thumbs together, squeezing the nipple between the thumbs, then pull outwards toward you. Do this until a complete circle is made around her nipple, adjusting the pressure based on her reaction. Repeat on the other breast.

Finally, during the "cooling down" phase of the massage, you will stroke and smooth her skin. Take the fingertips of both hands toward the center of one breast and radiate them from the center outward toward the side. Do this, at least ten times, and then repeat on the other breast.

The breast massage ends the same way it began, with one hand on her heart and the other on her Yoni, visualizing warm energy moving from your heart into your hands and down into her heart and Yoni. Breathe deeply and slowly together for several minutes, and then allow her to rest.

While the primary purpose of the Tantric breast massage is to please the receiver, it is enjoyable for the giver too. It is not only emotionally and physically healing, but it provides relaxation and a sensuous form of foreplay. It can be done alone or as the introduction to other Tantric massages such as the Yoni massage, clitoral massage, or G-spot massage.

The G-Spot

The G-spot (Grafenberg spot) is a tiny lima-bean shaped region located on the front (tummy-side) wall of the Yoni, two to three inches beneath the pubic bone. This area is different in texture than the rest of the Yoni, in that it is spongier and coarse. G-spot stimulation causes intense orgasmic feelings that are greater than in a normal sexual response.

How to Give a Tantric G-Spot Massage

In Tantra, the G-spot is known to store creative sexual energy, but also has another side; it stores sexual or emotional pain as well. Therefore, the G-spot massage, when performed correctly, can be healing as it can remove blocks to sexual pleasure, replacing them with positive sensations.

Once the receiver of the massage is undressed and lying face down, begin by giving her a ten-minute full-body massage. Once she is fully relaxed, ask her politely if you may massage her more intimately. If she obliges, gently massage her pubic area including the lips of her Yoni with high-quality lubricant.

Upon arousal, whisper in her ear that you are going to put your fingers inside of her. Lubricate your first two fingers well, insert them as far into her Yoni as is comfortable for her, and move them in even circles all around. Keep in mind that consistent, firm pressure along the entire length of the vaginal walls normally feels best, but you'll have to take her physical and audible cues as guides, as every woman is unique in her preferences. As a tip: pressing the palm of your other hand on the top of her pelvis can be very "grounding" for her.

Envision the G-spot as a clock. Spend a little bit of time with your fingers at each position of the clock. Pay attention to which "hours" feel best, which are numb, which may be painful, and which trigger some emotional reaction. If you find a great spot, press gently and hold. If any strong emotions arise such as anger, sadness or laughter, gently encourage her to describe anything she feels or "sees". Allow the energy to discharge, for this release of energy is healing and makes her sexual energy more available.

As the massage develops, begin to concentrate on pleasing her rather than on the numb or painful places. Another great way to stimulate the G-spot is by using the "press-and-release" technique:

1. Hook your fingers, pulling the G-spot upward.

2. Rhythmically press and release.

When the G-spot massage is finished, tell her that you are going to remove your fingers. As you gently slide your fingers out of her, press the mound of her vagina with your free hand, thus sealing the end of the Tantric G-spot Yoni healing process.

As a word of caution, it is important not to have any expectations regarding the outcome of this massage. Results may not be immediately visible and it may take a few tries before any emotions arise. In the meantime, take pleasure in becoming more familiar with your partner's Yoni and building a stronger bond between the two of you.

G-Spot Orgasms

Two conditions must be met to stimulate the G-spot. First, the woman must be aroused and secondly, pressure must be applied on the upper vaginal wall. Blood rushes to the G-spot similarly to how it does to the clitoris when a woman is sufficiently aroused, thus, any sexual position which places pressure on the area leads to greater chances of the woman experiencing the orgasm.

The Male Body

The Lingam (Penis)

"Lingam" is the Sanskrit word for the penis and is literally translated to mean "wand of light". In Tantra, the Lingam is viewed with respect and honored as a wand of light that channels energy and pleasure. Orgasm may offer a pleasant side-effect to receipt of a Lingam massage, but it is never the goal. The goal is to massage the organ, encouraging a man to relax and surrender to a deeper form of pleasure that he may not be used to.

Men must learn to relax and receive pleasure that is not goal (orgasm) oriented, as is common with traditional sexual expectation.

Taoist belief holds that the Lingam has reflex points similar to those in the feet or hands which when stimulated properly can affect the whole organ, allowing the massage to be both healing and sexual simultaneously. Applying pressure to different pressure points in the Lingam disperses energy to the entire body, leading to a wave-like experience of pleasure. This energy is dispersed all over the body, and then is built upon. In this fashion, men are able to experience full-body orgasms, and this wave of pleasure can last for a much longer time than a regular orgasm.

How to Give a Tantric Lingam Massage

Prepare a quiet dim space with a bed, futon, or a blanket and pillows on the floor. Make sure that the temperature is slightly warmer than normal, as you will both be nude. Lighting candles is an excellent idea both for lighting and temperature regulation. Your high-quality oils and lubricants should be within reach. Using spill-resistant bottles and plastic instead of glass is advised. And most of all make sure that you have a few hours of uninterrupted time so that you won't feel rushed.

Begin by standing or sitting face-to-face, and breathe deeply together. Touch each other by embracing or holding hands while looking into each other's eyes, breathing rhythmically from the belly. If he begins to hold his breath or lose focus, position one hand on his lower belly, and encourage him to breathe from that place and "fill his belly" with breath.

Have him lie face down and give him a full-body massage for at least ten minutes. Request that he turn over, and then continue his massage. Advance the massage toward the inner thighs and pelvis until his entire body is relaxed.

As a show of respect for his male power, ask for permission to touch his Lingam. If he is familiar with Tantric terminology, ask "May I touch your Wand of Light"? Otherwise asking "May I touch your Lingam?" or "May I touch your penis?" will suffice. If he obliges, cover his Lingam and testicles with the oil or lubricant. Rub the solution into his skin, starting at the top of his inner thighs, moving into the crease where his legs meet the pelvis. Release tension as you work along the connecting tissue, bone and muscles using slow, steady motions.

Continue by massaging above the Lingam on the pubic bone. Place one hand over this area, feeling the bone beneath the muscle. Slowly work your way down to the scrotum, very gently pulling on his testicles. It is important to pay attention to his physical and audible cues, as well as encourage him to let you know what feels right to him, as some men are averse to testicular pressure, while others very much enjoy stronger handling. Begin gently and slowly build pressure until you find the perfect amount.

Finally, slowly place one hand on the Lingam with your right hand. As you massage the shaft, squeeze the Lingam at the very bottom with your right hand, pull up, and slide completely off. Then alternate hands. Repeat this motion with each hand several times, and then switch direction -- slide alternating hands from the top back down to the base.

Take the Lingam between both hands and rub your hands together quickly as if attempting to start a fire. Hold the Lingam by the head and gently shake back and forth. Massage the head, cupping it in your palm and turning your wrist as if juicing a lemon.

If at any time he seems close to ejaculation, slow your movements and let him "cool down" before continuing. If he is close but not past the point of no return, you may be able to delay ejaculation by squeezing the tip of the Lingam between the thumb and forefinger very firmly and holding it for about thirty seconds, encouraging him to take deep breaths the entire time.

If you are successfully able to hold back his orgasm six times, tons of sexual energy will be stored. He can then retain and circulate this energy throughout his body, or choose to release. If he does choose to ejaculate, a much more intense orgasm than usual will be experienced. Remind him to take deep, controlled breaths as he ejaculates. Once the massage is complete, tell him that you will now remove your hands and allow him time to relax and enjoy the mind-blowing pleasure he has received.

The Testicles

Testicle massages can infuse the testicles with blood and clear out any blockages. Massaging the testicles on a regular basis can improve erections, ejaculation volume, and sperm count. The massage even has the potential to increase testicular size, making them fuller-feeling, lower-hanging, and more sensitive.

How to Give a Tantric Testicle Massage

Testicles are the most sensitive part of most men's' bodies, as such, many women fear massaging the area for fear of causing pain. The irony behind this is that it is exactly this sensitivity that incites pleasure once the area is stroked. The testicles can be one of the most erogenous spots on his body if stimulated properly, and a good testicle massage can be an outstanding experience for a man if a lover is doing it.

Once a safe, warm, ambient place is set and your man is comfortable and ready, here are eight steps that you can try to give a pleasing Tantric testicle massage:

1. Trace circles around the base of the penis where the shaft is attached to the scrotum.

2. Very lightly pinch the scrotal skin, gently rolling the skin between your fingers, and monitor his response.

3. Very lightly run your fingernails across the skin of his scrotum, paying close attention to his reaction. Some men absolutely love this sensation while others become nervous. If he likes it, continue. If not, stop.

4. With a firm grip, wrap your hands around his penis. Slide one hand up over the head and the other down across the testicles. This motion makes the penis feel big, expanding the sensation.

5. Cup the testicles and give them a gentle squeeze. Monitor his reaction, making sure that you aren't squeezing too hard.

6. Placing your hand at the bottom of the testicles, run your fingers from the bottom of the scrotum all the way up to the head of the penis in one smooth motion.

7. Hold the penis up, exposing the testicles, and tap them lightly with your middle finger.

8. Hold the penis and testicles in between the thumb and forefinger of one hand. Pull them both forward with your hand. Do this at least ten times in each direction -- up, down, left, and right.

Chapter 5: How to Give an Erotic Massage to Help Increase Intimacy

There are many different ways to give a Tantric massage and in time you will learn how to develop your OWN massage techniques suited to you and your partner. However, if you are confused as to how to begin, here is a guide, or rather two, on how to give your partner a sensual, Tantric massage:

Before you attempt how to learn to give a tantric massage, you have to take care of the ingredients you will be using. Learn them, put them together in the right combination and you will see your partner being very happy indeed. A Tantric massage delivered well and good can be one of the greatest doorways to passion.

Set the Mood

This is an extremely important part of tantric massage. This massage is supposed to be sexy and that will not be possible unless you are both into it. The best way to get into a situation is by setting the atmosphere or the mood of the room at a level of ease at which you are both able to indulge and lose yourself.

There are many ways you can set the mood. Try to alter the lighting by making it dim but not too dark. This provides a comfortable ambiance and will help your partner believe that their body looks sexy in the semi-darkness. Next, prepare the station. You will do this according to the type of massage you will be attempting to give. If it is a simple head or shoulder massage, you only need a chair. Otherwise it would be nice to prepare a stable surface such as a table or even the floor. Just remember that the surface needs to be firm enough for them to lie down so you can work your magic.

Music

This is an essential part of setting the correct mood for the massage. Note that in these situations, rough music such as heavy metal won't work. Choose something according to what your goal is. Sometimes you might want to give a massage to get them in the mood for sex and others you might want them to relax and drift off to sleep. Choose accordingly. If you are going for sex, choose something like intimate soul music. If you are going for relaxation, choose soft blues or nature sounds. Running water is especially soothing to help someone drift off.

The Oil

This is the vital ingredient for your massage. Consider this your turkey to your thanksgiving dinner. There are several different oils you can use, such as avocado, jojoba and grape seed oil. Experiment with a few and find what you like or what suits your partner the best. These oils are all usually available at health food stores, spa shops or skincare stores. You can even buy pre-blended massage oils that contain two or more oils. Make sure to buy any oil that helps your hands glide easily without chafing your partner's skin. Remember, comfort is the most important part of the whole massage.

Try and buy organic oil in small quantities and then store it in a cool and dry place.

Tantric Massage Techniques

This part will consist of two separate methods, one that will help you massage a female body and the other that caters to a male body's needs of the same. Fundamentally, both bodies are more or less the same but their treatment is somewhat different. Hence, here is the correct way to massage a female body:

Of course massages vary from type to type but one of the best tantric massages is the full body massage because it helps a person to relax under your touch and increases intimacy between you both.

Try and practice the techniques that are about to be relayed to you on your own body so that you know that you aren't being too hard on your recipient as well. Your thigh should be perfect to practice on.

Shiatsu

This is one of the easiest and most commonly used massage techniques in Japan. If you have received a massage with someone rubbing the knots under your skin out using their thumbs or elbows, you have had the shiatsu style massage treatment.

The technique involves placing your fingers or hands upon a particular place on her body. Apply gentle pressure and then move your hand or finger in a circular motion. The best spot for using this technique is the upper back, so use it to loosen up the knots in that area. Just make sure that you don't compress so hard that you cause her pain!

You might have seen experienced massage therapists applying pressure by using their elbows. However, this is an advanced technique that you should avoid unless you have real experience or are a licensed masseuse.

Compression

Compression is another popular method for massage. In order to perform a compression massage, you must apply pressure to one area of your partners' body. This will increase the flow of blood to this area and remove tension and rigidity from the muscle. This massage is much like a warm-up for the more intense styles of massage such as shiatsu. If you are extremely tense, don't go for shiatsu immediately because its intensity might injure you. Instead, have your partner give you a compression massage, it will boost blood flow and loosen up your muscles for shiatsu.

Stroking

The name of this massage is very descriptive. Stroking massages are very different from compression or shiatsu massages in that applying concentrated pressure does not perform them. Instead, this massage involves sliding your hands across parts of her body such as her thighs or back. It is a very stimulating form of massage and become extremely erotic if you do it right. It is also minimal in its intensity and a lot easier to do than compression or shiatsu massages.

Friction

This is a high-level technique that can be applied to the more bonier parts of your partners body such as her hands or feet. In this technique, you do not need to use oils. Instead, you must use your dry hands to generate heat via friction. The strokes must be firm but no hard, as compression is not required. In fact, compression would an impediment to the speed at which your hand is traveling across her body. This type of massage is in many ways a more advanced technique than stroking.

Kneading

This massage is amazing for reaching into deeper parts of her muscles and is especially good for relieving tension from the fleshy areas such as the buttocks. Be very gentle because you do not want to harm her. Do not perform this massage on her stomach because that will make her feel uncomfortable.

If you have ever baked bread before, you will realize that this massage is similar to kneading bread. To knead the muscles, take hold of the muscle and give it a slight dig with your fingers whilst raising the tissue with your thumbs. Do not lift too high because that will hurt. First, you will press your palm into their muscles, and then you will squeeze their muscles slightly and then give a gentle lift with your thumb. Try it gently on your thigh and use the same gentle motions on her skin. This massage is also good for her shoulders especially if you sense a tension in them. Remember to give her a little Shiatsu first, however, since directly kneading an already tense shoulder or neck muscle can be quite painful.

These massages are excellent if you combine them. Mixing up shiatsu, oil massage, compression, stroking and friction can be a great way to keep things interesting. Remember, doing the same thing over and over again will get boring for the both of you and will stop being effective after a little while, so apply different massage techniques to different parts of the body and your lover will be in heaven by the time you are done.

Tantric Massage for Males

The tantric massage for a man will be different than the normal erotic massage. Remember that a man might be more wary of a massage than a female though he may not show it. Put your partner at ease before you initiate this massage because you will be touching them in a way that might seem too intimate to their masculinity, hence be prepared to be gentle without seeming like you are patronizing them.

If you wish to massage your partner's penis, it is highly recommended that you use some kind of oil to make it easier to rub. Massaging a dry penis can result in chafing and is usually not nearly as enjoyable as a massage that is performed with oil. Using oil in this manner will also prevent you from potentially injuring your partner during the act of massaging.

A good massage that involves tantric practice would require the use of both of your hands. This is because you have several areas that you would ideally have to stimulate, and stimulating at least two areas at the same time will greatly boost the amount of arousal that your partner experiences.

Try to stroke his penis up and down whilst simultaneously massaging his testicles. His testicles are extremely sensitive, which means that if you gently stimulate them he is going to feel a ticklish and warm sensation within his penis. This will make him feel as though he is perpetually about to have an orgasm throughout your massage!

Chapter 6: Unlocking Intimate Capacity Through Synergy

The best lovemaking experiences come when you and your partner are moving and flowing in harmony with one another. Perhaps you have experienced this for yourself. What is the best sexual experience you've ever had? No matter what "type" of sex you had or with whom, it is likely that you and your partner were embodying the same energy and matching one another's passion. Whether you had rough sex, slow sex, sleepy sex, or spontaneous sex, the best sex comes from a perfect synergy between you and your partner.

The unfortunate thing is that we don't always know how to create this synergy; it just happens. The right environment, the right mood, the right time of day, and some other accidental factors often contribute to our most mind-blowing sex.

The heart of the Tantric sex practice is learning how to intentionally create the right elements to have the deep, intense, mind-blowing sex that everyone craves. In the last chapter, we learned how to set up one's physical environment to stimulate the senses and nurture deep intimacy. Now we will look at the internal factors that contribute to amazing, long-lasting, and profoundly fulfilling sex.

What is Energy?

Perhaps the most important aspect of Tantric practice is the energy that you and your partner bring into the experience. Without the right energy, all your setup and foreplay won't be nearly as effective in contributing to the overall Tantric experience. Setup and foreplay can certainly aid you in establishing the best energy for sex, but to get it just right, more intentional energy work is needed. True Tantra is much more about energy than about sex, wherein the focus is on merging the energies within yourself and then merging your united energy with that of your partner.

So, what is energy? Energy is the animating force behind all of the creation. It is what causes the movement of atoms, the formation of matter, and the evolution of life. Beyond the realm of the physical, energy is what composes the soul or spirit. It is what connects us to the center of divine creation itself.

When we talk about our energy, we are in part talking about the electromagnetic field that surrounds all bodies and the electric force within that animates our bodily functions. However, our energy is also composed of the spirit within our bodies, which is also made of energy.

Energy can take different forms. You may hear people talk about "good" and "bad" energy, or "positive" and "negative" energy. What they mean by this is that the emotions and intentions of which others "send out" their energy. When someone performs an action with kind and loving intentions, people say that they have "good" energy, whereas when someone does or says something that is fueled by anger or is meant to be hurtful, we say they have "bad" energy.

When we talk about people "sending" energy, we are discussing the actions, emotions, thoughts, and intentions that they manifest. While raw energy is essentially neutral, our thoughts and emotions can "bend" or "tint" our energy to match the tone of those thoughts and emotions. Others can pick up on our energy and interpret our intentions based on what they perceive. Hence, when people say that they will send us "good vibes" or "healing energy," what they mean is that they will have loving and positive thoughts about us and wish us well.

Energy is a complex force that can be used and interpreted in many ways. Since energy is the raw force behind all of the creation, we use energy in its purest expression when we create. We often do this unconsciously, allowing our reactive natures to determine what energy we put out into the world. However, when we start to become aware of our own energy and watch our thoughts and actions more carefully, we gain the power to choose the energy that we send into the world, which, in turn, determines what energy we are most likely to receive from others.

How to Recognize Energy

To reach a full understanding of what energy is and how to recognize and control it, you can start to practice in two different ways. First, you will learn how to recognize the electromagnetic field around your own body and that of your partner. From there, you will start to work with recognizing the energy around you as it manifests from others' thoughts, emotions, and intentions.

Learning to recognize your electromagnetic field is very simple, but it will take practice to get good at it. To begin, rub your hands together vigorously. You will start to feel the heat generated between your palms as the friction warms your skin. After a few moments, slowly begin to pull your hands apart, holding them just far enough apart that the skin of your palms is no longer touching. You will continue to feel the heat you generated by rubbing your hands together, as well as a slight tingling sensation.

Slowly begin to pull your hands further apart until they are about a half-inch away from one another. If you can still feel the warm, tingling sensation of your electromagnetic field, then you can move your hands to an inch apart. If you lose the feeling, move your hands closer together and start over.

Continue the exercise by pulling your hands further and further apart. If at any point you lose the tingling sensation, bring them closer together and move slowly apart again. Feel free to start over as many times as you need. The goal is to be able to sense the energy between your hands even when they are a foot apart or more. Advanced energy practitioners learn to shape and move energy for healing, but that is another line of study beyond what we will learn with Tantra.

You can begin to move your energy awareness to the rest of your body with another simple exercise. Bring your attention to one of your forearms, focusing as much as you can on the surface of your skin. When you are fully aware of your forearm, pull your attention to a quarter of an inch above your arm. If you can feel a sensation at that distance, you have found your energy field. If not, return your focus to your skin and begin again.

Like the hand exercise, you will continue to pull your focus farther and farther away from the surface of your skin. If at any point you lose your sense of your electromagnetic field, go back and begin again. Researchers have found that our energy fields extend an average of 10-15 feet beyond our physical bodies, so you can take this practice quite far before you will reach the edge of your energy field.

If understanding and sensing our own energy is difficult, learning to sense the energy of others is a much more complex matter. Knowing the energy of the people around us comes from a number of factors. Most of us begin to learn to recognize others' moods and reactions from their body language, the tone of voice, and facial expressions at a very young age. This innate sense certainly plays a role in our ability to sense the energy of others, though true energy awareness goes much further than that.

As you grow your awareness of your own energy field, you will slowly begin to feel when other people's energy fields collide with your own. If the sensation is pleasant or neutral, then you know that those people have "positive" or "neutral" energy that is in harmony with your own. If the feeling makes you uncomfortable, then that person likely has "bad" energy.

Another major part of learning to read others' energy is by developing your intuition. We can often tell what others are thinking or feeling in spite of their physical cues, especially our loved ones. We can't always explain these feelings; we just "know." This knowing, otherwise commonly referred to as a "gut feeling," is our intuition.

Accepting and trusting your intuition is the first step in developing it. The easiest way to validate your intuition is to practice with your loved ones. If you feel that you are picking up on emotions beneath the surface when talking to a friend or family member, ask them if anything else is going on. People often acknowledge their true emotions when prompted, even when they feel the need to keep them hidden in general.

You'll encounter plenty of other opportunities to develop your intuition as you go through life.

Sometimes you'll have an intuition to drive or walk one way instead of another or to choose one line at the bank or grocery store over the others. Learn to follow these feelings and great things will very often follow a pleasant conversation, an interesting find, or even the avoidance of some sort of accident. Your intuition is a powerful part of yourself that can aid you in many aspects of life, and it introduces an interesting element in the sexual experience for those who work to develop it.

Using Energy to Deepen Sexual Pleasure

Cultivating an awareness of your energy and your partner's will enable you to harmonize and channel your energies to create a smooth flow through your sexual experience. When both participants focus their intentions on creating a loving, open, and sensual, sexual encounter, the results can be astounding.

The first step to synchronizing your energy with your partner is to communicate openly about what kind of experience you both wish to have. If both partners want a different kind of sexual encounter, it is best to compromise so that both feel their needs are met. It is better to speak openly about what you want and what makes you uncomfortable rather than to see your desires collide mid-experience.

When you have agreed upon the type of sexual experience you both want, you and your partner can spend a few minutes setting your mutual intentions at the beginning of your ritual. Including intentions such as, "To have a healthy and nurturing experience together," "To achieve great emotional and sexual healing together," "To give each other the maximum amount of pleasure possible in an open and safe environment," or "To deepen our bond and create an experience that will make us feel closer to one another," are all appropriate intentions.

When establishing the energy for your sexual experience, it is crucial that both partners agree to only engage in sex if it is mutually wanted. Sometimes we get so busy in our lives that we need to schedule our intimacy to fit around our other obligations. However, when the time and day come, we might be too tired or stressed to feel like engaging sexually. Often, an argument or misunderstanding will create tension with our partners and we might not feel like sex is the best thing to do while there is discomfort between us.

If these situations should arise, it has to be okay for you to honor one another's feelings and not pressure each other into sex. You could agree to have a non-sexual Tantric session, where you will just massage and pamper one another, or you could talk through your issues or enjoy some other healing activity together. If both people are not completely on board with having sex, it is best not to compromise the integrity of your energy by trying to push forward.

However, if both people are completely ready and willing, you can harmonize your energies for the sexual experience by both showing up in a happy and loving mood. Allow yourself to feel all the love, compassion, and devotion to your partner at the start of your ritual. By opening the Tantric session with the right energy, you will ensure that you will both have the best sexual experience possible.

The Masculine and Feminine Aspects of the Self

Many of us are familiar with the concept of duality: for every state, there is an opposite. For every light, a dark; for every night, a day; for every hot, a cold; for every negative, a positive. The masculine and feminine are fundamental aspects of dual nature that are present in all of the existence. However, whereas philosophies of duality hold that these polar opposites usually remain separate, even when they meet, in Tantric philosophy, all opposites merge into one.

Everyone, whether men, women, or non-binary individuals, hold both masculine and feminine aspects within their beings. The masculine and feminine have less to do with one's gender than within the traits that one embodies. Some people have more masculine traits, while others have more feminine—and then there are those who have a nearly equal balance of both.

The masculine is assertive, active, direct, hard, linear, and focused. It is also associated with the aspects of light, heat, dry, and positive. The feminine, on the other hand, is passive, still, indirect, soft, circular, and abstract. It is associated with the aspects of dark, cold, wet, and negative. Whereas the masculine is the penetrating force, the feminine is receptive. The masculine bestows the seed of creation, while the feminine provides the ground for the seed to grow. The masculine is protective while the feminine is nurturing.

While everyone has the capacity for all these traits, some people embody more from one side of the spectrum than the other. When this happens, an imbalance might be present, and it is time to work on restoring harmony between the different aspects of the self.

How to Balance and Unify Your Masculine and Feminine

You may have observed many of these traits within yourself. Certain situations may evoke your more masculine traits, while others evoke your feminine. Many people naturally lean more one way than the other, usually in the direction of their physical gender. However, when an extreme imbalance is present, the effects can be harmful to the individual and those in their lives.

When there is an imbalance of masculine energy, people often become overly aggressive, confrontational, and hostile. The shadow side of the masculine is its tendency to pick fights and engage in ego battles. People with too much masculine energy can be egotistical and narcissistic, often bullying others into getting their way and refusing to listen to others. At its worst, the shadow masculine can be abusive and controlling.

A feminine imbalance, on the other hand, can lead individuals to be overly passive. These people refuse to assert their needs, to stand up for themselves, or to make things happen in their lives. They can be sensitive to the point that they can barely function, and they may listen to what others need more than working to meet their own needs. They can be scattered, unfocused, and messy. The worst of the shadow feminine is a tendency towards victimhood and martyrdom.

Balancing the masculine and the feminine is a necessary process that takes time and effort. When both aspects of the self are in balance, however, the individual can experience peace, harmony, and health within.

The first step to creating balance is to recognize where there are imbalances. Did either of the above descriptions resonate with you? When you identify which areas you need to balance out, then you can begin to cultivate aspects of the other energy.

For instance, if you are imbalanced in the direction of the masculine, you may be overly aggressive and independent, refusing to accept help from others, even when you need it the most. To correct this imbalance, you'll have to cultivate your feminine traits of patience, cooperation, and receptivity to allow yourself to slow down and include others in your endeavors.

On the other hand, if you have a feminine imbalance, you might be too dependent on others, too passive, and unable to get things done on your own. In this case, you would have to cultivate the masculine traits of independence and assertiveness to push through your obstacles and do what needs to be done.

Once your masculine and feminine energies are balanced, then you can begin to work on unifying them. Inner union comes when you accept all aspects of yourself and allow them to manifest in your life naturally. This could be particularly difficult for some who have learned that embodying one type of energy is "dangerous." For instance, people with a masculine imbalance may have learned at an early age that showing emotion and becoming vulnerable will only get them hurt, so they have become overly defensive and emotionally unavailable to compensate. Others may have been punished earlier on for asserting themselves and decided that being overly passive was a safer course of action.

As an adult, you have the power to write a new story for yourself and to build a life that makes it safe for you to embrace and embody all parts of yourself. It is only through full acceptance that you can unify your aspects within. Once you are whole, you can bring your wholeness forward in your lovemaking practices.

Enhancing Your Lovemaking with Masculine and Feminine Energy

Tantric sex holds the potential for significant healing in its capacity to promote the balancing of the masculine and feminine energies. The best sex comes when both partners are able to take turns embodying the masculine and feminine elements of sexual union. This allows you to switch roles and practice holding space for both energies through your lovemaking in a safe and open environment.

The partner embodying feminine energy will be relaxed, receptive, and open to being acted upon. Regardless of gender, either partner can play this role while the other is embodying the masculine role of acting. When you are in your feminine energy, you'll be receiving the attentions of your partner as they massage, caress, kiss, and please you. Nurturing your partner during lovemaking is another way to embody the feminine. If you communicate verbally during sex, listening to what is being said and being open to meeting the needs of your partner is a very healing way to embody the feminine.

When embodying the masculine, you will be assertive and active. You will be the one giving foreplay while your partner relaxes and receives your affections. Any time you speak up to assert your needs, whether you want to try something different or communicate to your partner that something is making you uncomfortable, you embody your masculine energy. If you take the dominant role in sex, for instance, taking the top position and moving your body to please your partner while they receive, this can be a very empowering embodiment of the masculine.

Understanding the masculine and feminine energies will allow you and your partner to take turns embodying them. When you consciously switch roles, you will see that it is safe to embrace both aspects of yourself and begin to heal and restore balance. This conscious switching will require you to slow down and allow both partners to act out different roles, which will extend your lovemaking and enhance your libido.

There is a world of pleasure available to those who are willing to be open to trying something new. By consciously working to balance your masculine and feminine energies through lovemaking, you will experience sex as you never have before.

Chapter 7: Spicy And Dirty Talk

She's eating a banana, but as she does, she peels back the skin and takes the banana into her mouth as if it's your dick. What she's trying to say is that eating a banana isn't what's on her mind. The language of dirty talk extends to body language. As her tongue goes over the top of that banana, she isn't thinking of fruit.

When he is rock hard and puts his hand upon your knee, he isn't after a cuddle. Sometimes you have to gage the ferocity of the language. If he's rock hard and ready, don't be a prude. Let him have what he wants and let him have it now. Drop your panties, sit on his lap and whisper dirty words into his ear.

The suggestive things that people do often get unnoticed. She dresses up especially for him but he's still got his mind on work. He brings her flowers but she's too busy on the phone talking to her friend. You need to re-introduce courtesies with your dirty talk. If you know you're in the mood, switch off the phones. If you know you want to catch him by surprise, make sure he's susceptible to it and relaxed. Often people misread the signals. She wants hot sex. He wants to recover from a day's work first. Let him unwind and use subtle dirty talk to see where that leads you. You may be surprised that the slowing down of the whole process actually puts all the obstacles out of the way and neither one of you has to be frustrated by the actions of the other – if forethought is put into the picture.

Walk past him while he's watching TV. Ask if he wants to fondle your breasts. If it's a man that is thinking in sexual terms, the best turn on for a woman knows that he thinks she's the hottest woman around. Drop a chocolate kiss onto her lips and then explore her body. "I can't wait babe, I need you right this moment, here and now." Hold her – let her know that she's the sexiest woman you know. If she says she hasn't got time or needs to be somewhere else, opt for a quickie because these can be every bit as much fun. Up close and dirty, move her to the edge of a table and reach up to take off her panties. "You want a quickie to keep you going until later?" may just get the reaction that you want. You know your woman. You have to be able to know what her response is likely to be. Hot, quick sex can really hit the spot sometimes while at other times passion, foreplay and after-play are so important.

Dirty talk adds suggestion. It also adds an element of excitement to your love life. "Get into that bedroom wench!" can make her wet on the spot if she is that way inclined. Grabbing him by the tie and leading him to the bed and telling him that you want what you want and are not giving in until you get it can get great results. You don't have to use the "F" word if that makes you uncomfortable, but you can still dirty talk in a subtle way that you both understand is meant to enhance your love lives rather than make them feel tacky and dirty.

Encourage your lover by telling him/her "Oh my, I love it when you do that with your tongue" because otherwise how will your partner ever know. "Do that again but a little to the left" helps him to find the place that really makes you go wild. "Show me what you're made of" is a taunt that will probably result in hard and horny sex. "I want to feel you deep inside me" will probably have similar results.

The problem is that often we are too busy making love to actually comment upon what's being done to us and that's a real shame. How does your partner know what you like? How does he know what you really don't like and what makes you cringe? Praise all those great moments because when you do, you let him know what pleasures you and since your pleasure is his main aim, he will do it more often because you voiced your opinion. That's vital to dirty talk.

Understand how all the different positions affect the depth of sex. If you don't want sex in the standard missionary position, tell him "I'm no missionary – move over mister" and roll on top of him for a change instead of letting sex become tedious. There are two people on the bed and the opinions of both count. "Hey that's so deep," tells him how effective his lovemaking is. Of course, he wants to hear that you feel he's large enough to pleasure you, so there's no harm in subtle dirty talk at all. It boosts his ego and it gets what you want more often.

A guy likes to have his ego stroked, but only if you are genuine. Try to avoid the obvious disaster words – words that are not specific to him or to her. A man who calls all women "darling" doesn't endear himself to his woman. It's not special enough because he uses it all the time and it's not specific enough to her. He could be talking to the girl at the local gas station. Think of horny names that are specific only to you. Similarly, when a girl cries out anything but his name, he's likely to feel a little irked by it. Some people even have randy bedtime names for each other that are hot and affectionate.

The reason I added this chapter was for those who are not accustomed to dirty talk and who are a little nervous about it. The introduction of dirty talk should start with you letting your partner know when something is so right it's pushing all the right buttons. You are complimenting your partner and how crude you want to be depends upon the way that the two of you are accustomed to talking to each other. Dirty talk doesn't have to be demeaning.

"I can feel your sperm squirting inside me"

"Make me cum with your hand!"

"Lick my clitoris until I am all hot and wet and ready for you."

These are words of encouragement. These are words that tell your lover what they are doing right and if you start with encouragement, you may find that you fall into talking dirty with each other simply because it leads on from what you are doing now – which is describing what you want to feel or what he makes you feel inside.

"Play dirty with me, make me cum" isn't something that you should be ashamed of. If he's started to turn you on and he knows that what he is doing is giving you such a lot of pleasure, he will be pleased to oblige. What women need to understand is that men need to be needed. They need to be adored in bed and they also need to acknowledge what they're doing. Otherwise, they may just as well be making love with a blow-up doll. When you both got together, you may have experienced other lovers, but that's not what it's about. Each lover that you have is a totally different, unique human being. By telling your partner what you feel, what you like and what he/she does to pleasure you, you open up avenues between you to develop that kind of lovemaking so that it's perfect.

It's actually quite endearing to know that the woman is the vamp in bed. That's something that she's good at, but remembers not to call her a "bitch" outside the bedroom because it's bad taste. You need to know the subtleties of the language of love and keep your dirty talk for when it's appropriate. Similarly, he isn't going to respond well at his mother's dining table if you reach your foot up to touch his penis. There are certain times when things are appropriate and times when they are not.

Knowing your partner well enough to know when it's appropriate to use dirty talk is important. There are times when it doesn't work because other things have the priority. Sometimes you both need the language of love and warmth, rather than the pleasure of hot sex with dirty talk, but if you vary your love making, you actually get the best of both worlds.

There's a lot to learn about what dirty talk is all about. Try it and don't knock it until you have. Your man may be very protective toward you, but he may also feel that sometimes it's nice that you take over and let him know what it is that pleasures you.

What women need to remember is that men and women out of bed have different approaches toward life. In bed, basically they want the same thing. Women hold back because they think they should. Men are gentle because they are protective toward their women, but when push comes to shove, a little variation in the bedroom can make the world of difference. If he wants you to be his "whore" in bed, then be it. Be brazen. Be brave and do things that have always been in your mind but you never actually had the guts to do. If she wants you to be masterful, take over. Tie her down to the bed and make her body writhe with pleasure. The language of dirty talk starts when you actually know that your partner accepts you for who you are – rather than who you have been behaving as because of society expectations. No one sees you in bed except him/her. It's a place where inhibitions can be dropped and you can experiment with all kinds of approaches.

If you want to eat strawberry yogurt from the end of his manhood, tell him. Give it your best shot and save a little so that he can have a similar experience in places you want him to explore. The language of love is one that two people can share and if they want to use dirty talk to help them get over the barriers that come between people then it's being used for a very constructive purpose.

Try a word game

Try to think up words that are juicy and sexy and have a contest with him to think of words to describe what it feels like when you cum. Try to think of words that make you horny or words that make you wet. Tell him. There's no shame in it and if you treat it as a game, then it's the prelude to something else. You have created a language of your own that you can pick up on at any time in the future and use to get your wicked way.

People talk about communication being one of the most vital things within a relationship and then get all prudish when it comes to suggesting dirty talk but all dirty talk becomes is an extension to other communication, but you communicate your sexual needs, wants and desires. What other thing can you think of that you can share with your partner that's more intimate, more special?

By exploring the world of dirty talk, you also explore something much deeper than that. You explore your sexuality. You teach your partner what pleases you and learn what pleases your partner. When you have great sex, you begin to realize that it doesn't have to be the same position – the same lead up to sex or the same rolling over and going to sleep after sex. Sex is much more than that. Teach your partner what you like, what you want and what you would actually enjoy and you open up a whole new dialog that helps your communication skills long after you have got out of bed. It's a dynamic to the relationship that is exclusively yours and that's extremely precious. "Make me wet. I want to feel all of you inside me in the shower" could be the start to a new day, and a whole new level of understanding.

Chapter 8: Masturbation

When the fantasy is allowed to flow naturally to the warmth of the hands through the body in search of sensations that lead to satisfying the desire, it is understood why no woman should give up masturbating; Not only for what it means of self-knowledge, but also because it greatly stimulates and deepens enjoyment. In that sense, renowned professionals in the field of medicine and psychology recommend autoeroticism as one of the most authentic and mature forms of sexuality.

Autoerotism awakens at a very early age and manifests itself in adolescence as an intense voluptuous tendency, leading to experiment with the body itself until knowing the hidden springs of sensuality that it ignites.

If self-stimulation is reduced to a simple sexual discharge alone, sexuality is impoverished, since masturbating is always pleasant. And it is not only a substitute for the lover, but it is also an intimate experience that relaxes tensions, avoids stress and contributes to personal serenity and balance. He also teaches and sensually prepares to guide the lover along the path of pleasure through his own body, complementing the erotic games between the two.

How to Enjoy it to the Maximum

A disturbing tickle that runs through the skin in sensual concentric waves that are not located in any area of the body, in particular, indicates to her the presence of desire. It could have caused a presence or a memory, the casual touch of soft underwear or a sentimental song, but whatever the reason, the fantasy begins to fly and gives way to the desire to find an intimate space to self-satisfy.

From that moment, the hands fly entangling themselves in the pubic hair, touching the nipples, crossing the tender line that divides the buttocks in two to reach the pink ring of the anus, and each rub is even more exciting and wakes up a thousand sensations at the same time. From the center of the body rises a heat that at times gains in intensity, the pores of the skin open releasing a thin layer of moisture and a liquid that lubricates it begins to flow, helping to slide the caresses.

The tension in the whole body increases. Little by little, the anxiety grows and, as it happens in all sexual practice, there is not just one unique technique to self-stimulate, but many. Each woman discovers that for herself and that is alternating or changing as you know better.

It is very pleasant to masturbate sitting just on the edge of a surface with your legs open, which allows you to caress the clitoris with one hand and with the other touch the breasts. The perception that intensifies by contracting the PC muscle and leaving the throbbing clitoris, traverses the entire vulva, and notice the sensations that occur in the vagina.

In Solitude

Her imagination is the maximum incentive to stimulate her libido, which makes masturbation one of the most exciting sensual experiences. Nothing prevents her from fantasizing that whoever is working her body has the most ardent and electrifying hands. Visualize your most ardent dreams while stroking, unleashes your excitement. Speak, groan, or scream with pleasure and you can even manage to realize that hidden or forbidden desire in your mind such as a sexual experience with more than one man or with a stranger, or to be taken with violence. You can also imagine risky places where to enjoy sex with the danger of being surprised and a thousand other things. She commands and decides on sexuality alone, is her own guide, her object of desire, and her source of self-satisfaction.

Taken by sensuality, she enjoys penis-shaped sex toys - the dildos - introduces them into the vagina while imagining that he hits her pelvis as she likes while rubbing the clitoris gasping with trembling longing. Images full of hedonism follow one another when a vibrator stimulates the anus or the vagina until it reaches the tense clitoris and its body moves sinuously with intense voluptuousness. Thus stimulated, she soon reaches the threshold of pleasure with her eyes wide open or her eyelids closed firmly rapid breathing, and her heart beating in a hurry until she reaches the pleasant orgasm.

In Couple

Masturbation between lovers is not only one of the games before penetration, but one of the most intense pleasure and probably the one that best contributes to self-knowledge. Nothing prevents her from fantasizing that whoever is going through her body and electrifying her are the hands of the man who excites her. She commands and decides on sexuality alone, is her own guide, her object of desire, and her source of self-satisfaction.

One of the many pleasurable positions to masturbate is to stand in front of a mirror or a fresh wall of tiles and scrub the burning body against it while stimulating the clitoris with one hand and the breasts with the other. Her hand crawls under her clothes looking for the pubis that opens the door to the center of pleasure.

When she is very excited, she begins to wish him to approach the key erogenous points and hint at it in a thousand ways or verbalize it directly, even while she is still dressed. His hand crawls under her clothes looking for the pubis that opens the door to the center of the enjoyment that they both crave. Between the wet hair of desire, he traverses the folds of the vulva with a finger, traces a tense and hot journey through the labia majora, and finally, finds the clitoris that beats anxiously waiting for contact. Her body moves to indicate what excites her most, wishing that the caress rotates, turns, rises, and descends looking for other high centers, while the tongue licks the breasts that she offers yearning.

When he continues to masturbate, she contracts the PC muscle and feels an intense pleasure that extends through the vagina until it climaxes, and if at that point he penetrates her, her orgasm will multiply and become several which will be transported in sensual waves through the whole body, satisfying their desire.

Chapter 9: Orgasms

The word orgasm comes from the Greek word *orgasmos*, which means excitement and swelling. An orgasm in the sudden discharge of accumulated sexual excitement during a sexual session. This discharge results in the rhythmic muscular contraction of the pelvic region and is often described as the height of sexual pleasure in that session.

Orgasm can occur during sex with a partner or during masturbation, and it involves the release of tension in the body. This combination of feeling often goes by many names such as climaxing, cumming, and coming. Orgasming is often characterized by involuntary actions such as muscle spasms, vocalizations, and a general feeling of euphoria.

There are different types of orgasms that a person can experience they include:

- *Tension orgasms.* This results from direct stimulation or results in the release of tension from the body and muscles when it occurs.
- *Multiple orgasms.* This occurs when a series of orgasms occur over a short period of time.

- *Blended orgasms.* This is also called a combination orgasms and results when different types of orgasms are experienced at the same time such as orgasms from oral stimulation and penetration.
- *G-spot orgasms.* These occur from penetrative intercourse and direct stimulation of the erotic zone.
- *Pressure orgasms.* These kinds of orgasms occur from indirect stimulation of applied pressure such as touching through clothing.
- *Relaxation orgasms.* These occur when a body is deeply relaxed during sexual stimulation.
- *Fantasy orgasms.* These result from mental stimulation alone.

There are many biological or physical responses that you will notice when a person orgasms. These responses include:

- Warmth and redness spread across the face and chest.
- Increased breathing rate.
- A quickly beating heart.
- Muscle spasms of the genital and lower abdomen.
- Tension in the thigh and back.

- A rise in blood pressure.
- Temporary loss of motor control.

An orgasm is not just a physical response; it also induces emotional and cognitive changes in the body. Emotional and psychological reactions include:

- Altered states of consciousness.
- Altered states of space and time.
- Activation of the reward pathways in the brain.
- Decrease and inactivation in mental regions associated with behavioral control, anxiety, and fear.
- Feelings of relaxation and happiness.

While these signs and symptoms are general for both males and females, both males and females have decidedly different biological responses to orgasms. Before we get to the characteristics of both male and female orgasms, let's take a moment to look at a few facts concerning orgasms:

- Orgasms have many great benefits apart from the release of sexual tension such as the reduced risk of prostate cancer, pain relief, and even an increased lifespan.

- Orgasms do not only occur during sexual stimulation and can result from everyday activities.
- Orgasms can occur with or without the presence of a condom, and the barrier does not hinder the occurrence of orgasms.
- Women find it harder to reach orgasm compared to men. Up to 40% of women report having difficulty or inability to reach orgasm during sexual stimulation.
- One of the best ways to stimulate a female to orgasm is through clitoral stimulation.
- The quality and frequency of orgasms can improve as women age.
- Self-esteem is a huge factor that influences the occurrence of orgasms during sexual intercourse.
- Women usually take more than 20 minutes to orgasm while it takes a shorter period of time for most men.

Male Orgasms

A male orgasm is only possible after a man gets erect as a result of excitement. Erection occurs when blood flows to the penis causing it to swell in size and become rigid. The testes also become drawn toward the male body. As a result of stimulation, a man's blood pressure will rise, his pulse will quicken, and his rate of breathing increases, all of which are symptoms that he is being sent closer to the ultimate fulfillment.

The act of a man orgasming is called a resolution. It is often thought that males have to ejaculate semen during an orgasm, but it is possible to have an orgasm without ejaculation. When a man does ejaculate during orgasm, he can squirt up to 2 teaspoons of semen, which is a white fluid that contains sperm and other entities.

After a man orgasms, there comes a temporary recovery phase where more orgasms are not possible. This is called a refractory period, and its length varies from man to man, ranging from a few minutes to a few days. Generally, this period becomes longer as a man grows older.

Female Orgasms

Excitement incites the possibility of a woman orgasming. When a woman is sexually excited, blood vessels within her genitals dilate to increase blood flow supply to that region. Her vulva becomes swollen and fluids are secreted from her vaginal canal making her "wet." Just like with a man, her heart rate picks up, high blood pressure rises, and her breathing quickens.

As a woman's excitement begins to plateau, her breasts will increase in size by as much as 25%, and her nipples will become erect. When an orgasm does occur, her genital muscles will experience rhythmic contractions that are less than one second apart. The female orgasm usually averages in length of about 13 to 50 seconds. Ejaculation is not a common symptom when a female orgasms, although it is possible and is sometimes called female ejaculation. It involves the squirting of a clear liquid that is commonly confused with urination, but it is not, and it is not something that a female should be ashamed of or embarrassed to share with her partner.

Women, unlike men, do not experience a refractory period and can have further orgasms if stimulated again.

Different People Orgasm Differently

No matter the symptoms or characteristics that you exhibit during orgasm, there is no right way or wrong way to reach that culmination of feeling. Some people can reach orgasm quickly and easily, while others need more time and stimulation to get to that point. Some positions work best for some, while others can orgasm strictly from penetration. Some people need masturbation or the aid of toys or visual stimulation. All of this and others are perfectly normal and perfectly fine. Go with what feels good to your body, and experiment to find the other ways that make you climax. A good, supportive relationship partner will encourage you to explore your body and its responses to different stimuli and put in the work necessary to bring you pleasure. In response, you should do the same.

As a final note, having an orgasm should not be the ultimate thought when it comes to having sex as it puts too much pressure on reaching that moment. This can make you and your partner anxious. This makes the act of sex stressful and definitely unfulfilling, especially if that ultimate goal is not reached. Relax and let the natural flow of things happen so that you and your partner get the most pleasurable response from sexual intimacy.

Sexual Positions to Incite Male Orgasm

While it is true that men find it easier to orgasm compared to women, there are sex positions that are guaranteed to completely blow his mind. These usually focus on stimulating nerve endings at the tip of his shaft and allow him to build up toward prolonged pleasure.

Prolonged Hand Job

In this instance, it is about making it completely about the man's pleasure. Have him lie down or sit in a reclined position that is comfortable for him while naked. Get between his knees and with a hand and fingers that have been well-lubricated start to stroke his engorged member. Start off by stroking slowly and slowly building strength and speed. Move your hands in an up-and-down motion. You can vary the length and strength of your motions while using one hand or both hands at the same time. If you are using both hands, twist your hands in opposing directions as you move up and down. If the man is circumcised, you can slide the skin of his shaft up and down for added sensation. If he is uncircumcised, move the foreskin back gently and tease the sensitive area just below the tip of his shaft.

Keep eye contact with him as you do this. To make this interlude as pleasurable as possible for the man, pull back or slow the strokes of your hand as you feel his body moving closer to orgasm so that you prolong the drive. This makes the strength of the orgasm stronger when it does finally come.

Do not be afraid to ask him if he likes what you are doing or to show you how exactly he wants the motions of your hand or hands to proceed.

The Sensual Panther

In this position, the woman lies on top and parallel to the man. Her chest and legs are pressed against him. The woman has the leeway of being able to stimulate him in different ways such as kissing along his neck and whispering dirty talk to him. Since her legs are not spread, the penetration in this position is shallow but tight and allows the man to last longer and build up slowly toward a powerful climax.

Turntable

In this position, the woman lies on her side with her legs brought to a 90-degree angle to her upper body. The man lies on top of her just as he would in the missionary position, but the angle of penetration is different since she is lying on her side and he is not between her thighs. This position is great for men because it promotes tightness and pressure around the penis. If the man's penis is curved to the left or right, there is the added bonus that it will stimulate the front or back of the woman's vagina.

Side by Side

This is a position that promotes shallow penetration and, therefore, is great for allowing a man to prolong his climax. In addition, it allows the partners to have lots of eye and skin contact, and so it promotes deeper emotional connections. To get into position, the partners need to lie facing each other. The man's pelvis needs to be slightly lower than the woman's. She will lift her top leg and wrap it around his waist. This position can be thought of as a back to front spoon. The woman may need to tilt her lower body away from the man's or lift her leg higher to allow penetration.

The Cross

In this position, the man lies on his side while the woman slides into a position perpendicular to his body. Her legs will be draped over his hips with her feet ending up behind his buttocks. She needs to press her pelvis against his and open her legs slightly to allow penetration. The man can aid thrusting by gripping the woman's hips and pulling her back and forth on him. He can also reach down to stimulate his partner's clit. This position helps the man last longer because his range of motion is limited and the penetration is shallow.

Modified Sitting in a Chair

In this position, the man sits in a chair and the woman sits on top of him with her back to his front. The woman gets more control in this sex position and can move up and down, grind her pelvis against the man and even use her PC muscles to squeeze his member to her leisure. This position works to prolong the man's pleasure because since the woman is in control, he cannot get carried away. He also has his hands free to touch other parts of her body.

Sexual Positions to Incite Female Orgasm

Women find it harder to orgasm from penetrative sex, but with foreplay and the right position, anything is possible. The sex positions that will be described below promote having the penis stroke the walls of the vagina as well as clitoral stimulation so that the woman has a greater change of climaxing.

Altered X Marks the Spot

This position is wonderful for women since it allows the man's penis to stimulate her G-spot when he penetrates her. This stimulation is facilitated by the upward pressure on her vaginal walls by the tip of the man's penis. To get into position, the woman lies on her back with her knees crossed and her knees brought up to her chest. Her pelvis is braced against the man's thighs and he is able to thrust into her. This position is great for the man, too, since the position requires her to have her thighs closed, which increases the tightness of penetration.

Linguini

To get into this position, the woman lies on her front with her body slightly tilted to one side with one leg slightly raised. The man gets behind her and puts one leg under her raised up so that their lower halves are scissored. This position is great for women since it not only allows the man to stimulate her G-spot with his thrusts but she can also have her clitoris stimulated by grinding against the man's thigh. The man benefits, as well, since the position promotes greater tightness around his penis.

Standing Delivery

In this position, both parties are standing. The woman is in front and faces away from the man. To align their pelvises, one party may need to bend their knees depending on who is taller. Once the pelvises are aligned, penetration can be achieved. This position is great for promoting female orgasm since the clitoris is easily accessed. The man can also play with other parts of the woman like her breasts and other erogenous zones in her front while being able to kiss her neck and lips if she tilts her head toward him. The man also can have an amazing orgasm since there is increased friction and tightness due to the angle of penetration.

Sitting Scissors

In this position, the man sits and the woman gets on top. She kneels with her back to his front and places one leg on the outside of the man's body and the other leg between the man's legs. She then fits her pelvis against the man's to allow penetration. Women find it easier to orgasm in this position because they can control the length and depth of penetration in addition to having their clit stimulated by themselves or by the man. The man can also increase the pleasurable sensations the woman feels by playing with breasts and kissing her neck and back. The man can also lie back to vary the depth and angle of penetration.

Sideways Straddle

This is a girl on top position. The woman kneels facing away from the man with her knees on either side on one of his legs. The man needs to raise this leg so that it presses against the woman's clitoris. The woman can use her hands to guide the man's penis into her vagina. Women love this position for the obvious clitoral stimulation as well as being able to control the intensity and depth of penetration.

Chapter 10: Sex Toys: What Choose For Him And For Her

The first sex toy I ever used was a dildo. After that, a trip to the sex shop for Valentine's Day started a couple month long foray into the incorporation of toys into my sex life. It's one of the best decisions I ever made.

They are not only a quick and efficient way to take your sex life to the next level, but they're super fun to mess around with. They can do things we simply can't do, or at least not as skillfully (like vibrate).

However, it's important not to think of them as REPLACEMENTS, but rather ENHANCEMENTS of you, your partner(s), and the sex life you already have together.

The name of the game is pleasure, connection, fun, and intimacy. Sex toys help with all of that. By themselves, they can only accomplish a mere fraction of it.

So for people who are hesitant to venture into the world of these devices because of an insecurity you have about them (like I had), trust me when I say it's completely unfounded and you are truly missing out on an exciting aspect of sexuality, not to mention you may be leaving your partner hanging.

There are a number of directions I could have gone with this chapter, but I decided to focus it purely on using sex toys while having sex itself. I also decided to focus on how to use them to optimize the pleasure of both partners.

There are TONS to choose from. It can be quite daunting the moment you step into the sex shop or the online store loads on your computer screen.

Dildos, vibrators, BDSM devices, masturbators, anal stimulators, dolls, edible underpants – the list goes on and on. And within each type of toy are different sub-categories meant for different pleasure goals. So how am I going to narrow this down?

I'm only going to go over the main ones. Why? Because once you understand how they work and have experienced them, that's when you gain a strong enough background knowledge to choose the ones that are REALLY going to enhance your experience.

You will also feel much more comfortable starting out with these than some of the more intricate ones. I've also included links to examples of each to give you a better idea of what I'm talking about.

Diddling Around with Dildos

Dildos are typically made out of a silicone, silicone-type material, or glass and have a phallic shape (the general shape of a penis).

It's a good beginner's toy because it's not complicated to figure out how to use it. If you have a penis, you already know how. Use it like you would your penis.

The following suggestions can be practiced as a part of foreplay, as a break from intercourse in the middle of a session, or whenever it tickles your fancy.

- If you're using a dildo on your partner and they haven't been penetrated yet, enter them slowly and be attentive to how they react. Using a good amount of lube is also recommended.

- Angle the toy towards the G-Spot and/or prostate for maximum pleasure. It can also be used to stimulate the clitoris and/or outer part of the anus or perineum as well.

- In the case of penetrative sex for those who have a vagina, dildos can be used for double penetration (stimulating the vagina with the penis, and the anus with the dildo) or the other way around.

- Strap-on dildos also fall under this category and can be used in any of the above ways.

- You can also find double-penetration dildos, which can be used to stimulate one partner or to be shared between two partners (be aware of hygiene concerns).

- Dildos can also have a vibrating component. The most common are "rabbit" vibrating dildos which have a protrusion from one side, meant to stimulate either the clitoris or the anus.

- There are also dildos meant for anal stimulation. The most common are referred to as "butt plugs," and have a splayed bottom so the toy doesn't get lodged inside the rectum.

Example dildos to check out:

- Glass Dildo with Ribbed Sides
- "Rabbit" Dildo with Vibration

Vibrators – Bite-sized Pleasure That Packs a Punch

Vibrators are usually made of plastic and generally come in smaller sizes. But these little Energizer Bunny sex toys pack a powerful punch.

For many, and those who have vaginas especially, the use of a vibrator is one of the only ways they can orgasm during intercourse. For some, this includes masturbation as well.

Either way, using vibrators is one of the best ways to enhance your sex.

- A torpedo vibrator comes in the shape of a miniature torpedo. They're about 2-4 inches in length and are one of the most common vibrators.
- Typically, vibrators have different settings that allow you to adjust the speed and intensity of the vibration.
- For those who have a vagina, focus most of your efforts on and around the clitoris. Pay attention to how your partner is reacting. When using a vibrator, the clitoris can become overstimulated rather quickly.

Stimulation above, to the side, and on the sensitive tissue below the clitoris might be more pleasurable for your partner.

- For those with a penis, using a vibrator on the head and/or testicles can be pleasurable as well.

- For anal play, focus vibration where the highest density of nerve endings are – the outer tissue, inner two-thirds, and the prostate or area close to the G-Spot.

- Vibrators truly stand out during sexual intercourse. As long as you are in a position where either you or your partner can reach a hand to a part of the other partner's genitals, vibrators can be used. For G-Spot or prostate stimulation, I have found that the best position is either missionary or the first position we described, "Missionary With Legs in the Air." During these positions, penetration is providing intense stimulation on the inner part of the genitals, so you can intensify the experience by using a vibrator to stimulate the outer part of the genitals.

Example vibrators to check out:

- Typical Torpedo Vibrator
- A Popular Type of Massage Vibrator
- Dual-Stimulation Vibrator

Vibrating Rings

Commonly called "penis rings," vibrating rings are just as their name describes – rings that vibrate. Don't worry, they're elastic and usually the part that vibrates is protruding outward.

- For penetrative sex, wearing the ring over the object that is penetrating can add pleasure for both partners.
- For the receiving partner, make sure the ring is positioned so it can make contact with your genitals as your partner thrusts. It should also make the entire penetrating object vibrate as well.
- As the penetrating partner, it's your job to control the stimulation. Rather than constant continuous thrusting, try slow and careful movements. Pause when you are all the way in and the ring has made contact with your partner. Allow the feeling to soak in. Then pull

out suddenly, and move in extremely slowly again, teasing your partner. They'll be dying for you to go all the way in. Make them crave it before giving it to them. Don't forget our old motto of give and take.

- You can also find tongue vibrating rings which are meant for cunnilingus. In my experience, they flat out suck, so I wouldn't spend too much money if you plan on buying one. It's an awesome concept, but the execution is awful. Using it is almost like performing cunnilingus while your tongue is numb, because you can't feel what you're touching. I wouldn't recommend it, but hey, maybe you will be more skilled than me.

Example vibrating rings to check out:

- Trojan Brand Vibrating Ring
- Classic Vibrating Ring
- Vibrating Tongue Ring

Kinky and Restrictive Devices

Constraint is a turn on for many people. It helps define and play out the sexual roles of domination and submission. However, a common complaint is one partner wanting to kink up their sex life while the other doesn't feel comfortable with it.

There are numerous psychological reasons behind this. But the bottom line is that you two should progress slowly, carefully, and supportively. Both partners need to have a high level of trust and must know when to stop before things go too far.

That being said, there are some fun introductory items to use that aren't too crazy and will still add an entirely new dynamic to your sex life.

- **Blindfolds**. Putting a blindfold on one partner can be extremely sexy. The partner that's blindfolded is suddenly engorged in a world of mystery, while the other is given the perfect opportunity to be creative. Their partner won't know what's about to happen to them until it happens. The partner without the blindfold should take this opportunity to tease them like crazy. Run your fingers up their body. Barely graze over their private parts. Make them crave knowing what's going to happen next. Then make it happen. Again, the level of trust must be high, but this is a great place to start.

- **Rope Ties**. As far as constraint goes, rope ties should be your first stop. You can tie up any appendages and restrict their range of motion. By doing this, you give your partner something to flex against while they're being stimulated, which can help them orgasm. There is also a lot of cognitive pleasure involved, as one partner submits control to the other. It's a fun way to play out certain fantasies. However, proceed with caution. Tying people up certain ways can cause injury.

- **Handcuffs**. These provide similar pleasure to rope ties, but the cognitive pleasure of being handcuffed is different from being tied up. Handcuffs are usually made of metal as well, which can be painful. Try to find a pair that has a cushiony or protective covering.

Example kinky and restrictive devices to check out:

- Padded Leather Blindfold
- Rope Tie and Vibrating Dildo
- Cushioned Handcuffs

Those are the main introductory toys that I decided to include. Of course, there are loads more. A quick Google search is evidence of that.

If you would like to check out more of what's out there, here are a few online stores:

- Adam and Eve
- <u>Spencer's</u>
- Pure Romance
- Amazon – Sex Toys Department

Look at sex toys as a way to introduce a kinkier side to your sex life. Challenge yourself to see just how high you can increase the pleasure of you and your partner. It's an interesting endeavor, and worthwhile once you take the plunge.

This next chapter discusses something that literally changed my sex life in one night.

Enough said.

Chapter 11: Using Props During Sex

The ideas in this chapter are just suggestions to start with. Feel free to experiment with your partner and find out what excites you both!

Props to Set the Mood

One very easy way to use props during sex is to use them to set the mood. A bedroom that is sensually decorated is a perfect reminder to you and your partner to save a little time for yourselves, and you can also use special decorations for times when you want to surprise your partner or have a particularly memorable evening. There are many different ways to use props to create the sexual atmosphere that you and your partner desire. Candles, in particular, are a nice way to turn an ordinary bedroom into a sexy boudoir. Scented candles can make the room smell wonderful, while the low lighting invites sexual advances. For those with a sense of humor, there are also fun, phallic candles that can be found online or at your local sex shop. Decorate to set the mood that you want to create!

Vibrators and Dildos

Many people may think that vibrators and dildos are for masturbation and not useful while having sex with a partner, but these toys can actually be a fun addition to a couple's sex life. Vibrators can be added in as a couple has penetrative sex, particularly in positions where the woman is able to stimulate her own clitoris. Many women have trouble achieving an orgasm with penetrative vaginal stimulation alone, so using a vibrator while having sex can help to ensure that she has just as much fun as he does. He can also use a vibrator on her as they have sex. Try using a vibrator during some of the positions in chapters 1, 2, and 3 of this book, such as Ride 'Em, Ladies and Puppy Love (Easy), All About Legs, Take a Ride in Reverse, and Keeping it Erect (Intermediate), and Come From Behind (Advanced).

Vibrators and dildos can also be a great addition to mutual masturbation. Some men find it difficult to provide intense enough stimulation to the clitoris with their fingers to bring a woman to orgasm. A vibrator can help in these situations. In addition, some women like the feeling of their vaginal opening being stretched very wide, even wider than most men's penises can physically get. Men shouldn't be offended by this, but rather treat it as an opportunity to use a dildo and get the woman very turned on before having penetrative sex. Some women like the feel of a dildo when it is inserted and does not move, while others like an in-and-out movement more similar to sex. Communication is key for unlocking the possibilities of vibrators and dildos!

Using Food as a Prop

Food is one of the best classic erotic props due to its availability and the endless possibilities that come with incorporating it into sex. It might be a little daunting to walk into a sex shop and purchase a vibrator, but it's not in the least difficult to go to your local grocery store and buy some whipping cream. If you and your partner are looking to mix up your sex life without getting too daring, using food as a prop is a perfect place to start.

One of the easiest ways to use food as a prop is to incorporate it into erotic massage and foreplay. Try covering your partner's body or sensitive areas with a creamy or spreadable food and then licking them all over until they are clean. You can use whatever food you prefer, but some easily used foods are whipping cream, chocolate syrup, marshmallow creme, peanut or almond butter, chocolate hazelnut spread, jams or jellies, and frosting. You might want to put down a towel beforehand or plan to change the sheets afterward!

Ice is one of the most flexible foods when it comes to sex. To avoid the uncomfortable sticking sensation of very cold ice on the skin, use "warm ice," which has been out of the freezer 10-20 minutes and is starting to melt. You can run ice cubes up and down your partner's body, concentrating on their erogenous zones. You can also put ice cubes in your mouth and then put your mouth on your partner's body, even during oral sex. This can produce very different and exciting sensations. It's also possible to insert ice cubes into a female partner's vagina. Just make sure to use warm ice when you do this since very cold ice can have sharp edges that can be painful.

Another way to incorporate food into sex is to feed one another. It's highly dubious that any foods (oysters, dark chocolate, ginger, or otherwise) actually affect libido, but some people are turned on by feeding a partner or by getting fed by a partner. The easiest way to try this is to start with easy-t0-eat foods in bite size pieces. Pieces of fruit, small chocolates, or nuts are a good place to start. Eating or feeding your partner too much of a heavy food may make you or them less willing to have sex since they may start to feel unwell, so be careful. Otherwise, find out what you and your partner like, and have fun!

One important consideration when using food as a prop during sex is to not insert any food into the vagina that may get stuck there. People certainly have used particular kinds of vegetables as dildos, but it's a lot safer just to go and buy a sex toy. A dildo made to be inserted into the vagina is unlikely to break off and get stuck there, unlike a carrot, for example. Vegetables are also organic matter and can carry bacteria that is not good for the vagina. The same is true for candies, which have the added problem of being very sugary. This sugar attracts unhealthy bacteria, which can lead to infections. In general, if you and your partner would like to insert an object other than a penis into the vagina, use a dildo, a vibrator, or ice, since it will simply melt into water rather than getting stuck.

Other Sex Toys

There is a huge variety of other sex toys that you and your partner can incorporate into your sex lives. Many of these toys can be found at a sex shop or online. A sex shop may be embarrassing to visit, but rest assured that there is nothing shameful about enjoying sex and using toys. By going to a sex shop, you can get a better idea of what a toy looks like and if it is good quality or not. Going online can be less stressful, but you run the risk of ending up with a poor-quality toy. When it comes to sex toys, it's always better to spend a little extra money to get a quality item. You don't want yourself or your partner to get hurt using a cheap toy.

Many sex toys are bondage-type toys that can heighten the excitement for couples, especially those who enjoy dominant/submissive sex play. Blindfolding your partner, handcuffing them, or tying them to the bedposts are all ways to incorporate this type of toy. You can find special blindfolds, handcuffs, and ropes for use during sex, which is a good idea because everyday versions of these items are not always well-suited for sex play.

Other sex toys are meant to add to the sensation produced by the penis during penetrative sex. The simplest of these toys are specialty condoms, which can usually be purchased at drugstores. These condoms have extra ridges, bumps, or textures, which can be fun for women. More specialized toys include penis extenders, some of which also include extra bumps and ridges, and strap-ons, which allow for a woman to penetrate a man anally. If you and your partner are interested in some of these more elaborate toys, it could be fun and sexy to visit a sex shop together and pick out a toy to use together. You'll both be looking forward to getting home to try it out!

A final consideration for all sex toys: make sure you are cleaning them well and not sharing them with others! Sex toys, especially those that penetrate the body, should be personalized. Sharing these toys could transmit infections, particularly STI's, so be careful, keep your toys clean, and stay safe!

Chapter 12: Sexual And Aphrodisiac Food

Choosing the right food is easy because every religion and every culture have their share of special food. One can choose from common vegetables and fruits like broccoli, artichoke, leafy greens onion, ginger, and eggplant. These help the juices flow. Here you will see some popular food items.

Eat the right foods

For having good sex that is satisfying you need to have a good flow both through your blood vessels and through your sex organs. You need to satisfy your sex fantasies, so eat well. Foods that increase the flow of blood, testosterone and estrogen are available from our grocery shop. Eating these types of fruits and vegetables will keep you in fit condition always. Your sexual intercourse will be vigorous and satisfying. Here are some of these "sexy foods".

Chocolate

Chocolate dates back a long way in history to the times of Casanova and Louise the XV in terms of being used for stimulating the passions. However, this is applicable only to dark chocolate or at the least containing 70% or more of dark chocolate. The magic ingredient in chocolate that helps boost your senses is phenyl ethylamine. Keep a few pieces in the back of the cupboard for those times when you are feeling low.

Horseradish

This food item is quite popular in Japan. People eat it with their sushi and this side dish packs a wallop in the excitation department. Check out the items in your nearest mall, you might get lucky.

Chili Peppers: This spice helps boost the metabolic rate, meaning it gets the blood flowing. This supposedly triggers the release of endorphins that puts you 'in the mood'.

Oysters: Famous since the olden ages as an aphrodisiac, oysters have zinc in them that is beneficial for the production of testosterone. This increases the sex drive in both men and women. Women get easily "into the mood" when they have oysters.

Nuts: Pine nuts help your libido. They are good for your brain too. Nuts like almonds have plenty of essential amino acids that help to keep sex hormones thriving. Brazil nuts will benefit men more because the selenium content will keep the health of the sperm cells intact.

Caviar: Caviar is fish eggs that have plenty of vitamins. Many people have a sex fantasy that involves caviar. It has phosphorus that makes your nerves steady and active. The best combination for caviar is vodka. But do not drink too much vodka, only a little, or you may have trouble maintaining an erection.

Avocado: Since the time of the Aztecs, avocados have been accepted as one major fruit that increases a person's vitalistic energy. The very shape of the fruit is sensuous and delicious; over the past few years, scientists have been studying how much of an aphrodisiac the fruit actually is. Despite the fact the research is still being conducted, the fact remains that avocado contains high levels of Vitamin E and helps you retain an energy level that is unprecedented.

Honey: The very idea of honey is something that sparks a sensuous image in our heads; not for nothing do we call sex 'the birds and the bees'. It has long since served as a symbol of procreation in literature and art, but the fact is adding a few spoons of honey to your daily diet will boost your sex life unimaginably! It contains the nutrient boron, which not only gives you a natural energy boost but also regulates your estrogen and testosterone levels, so use honey creatively in food as well as your lovemaking!

Pine Nuts

Doctors, having studied these little gems over years, suggest that pine nuts are incredibly helpful in maintaining an active and healthy sex life. This is because they are rich in zinc, which is a highly energizing mineral that leads to a powerful sex drive. Just extracting these nuts from pinecones is hard enough, so be sure to add it to your diet to boost your sex life!

Arugula

This exotic sounding plant is a food that has been documented as an aphrodisiac since early times. It contains a host of minerals and antioxidants; like a number of its other leafy green counterparts, this plant counters the effects of any toxic substances that your body has absorbed from the environment that kills your libido. It boosts your immunity, thereby increasing overall energy levels and vitality.

Olive Oil

Not only is olive oil a much healthier option to cook with, it helps with your sex drive as well! It is rich in antioxidants and is an excellent source of both monounsaturated as well as polyunsaturated fats – these fats keep your blood flow pumping, your heart healthy and aid in the regulation and production of hormones too! The Greeks believed that olive oil makes men that much more virile; whether this is true or not is still under research, but the fact is that it increases overall energy and boost vitality, which is always brilliant for a healthy sex drive!

Pomegranates

Looking sensuous and exotic from the get go, pomegranates are some of the most nutritious fruits around. They are rich in antioxidants and support a powerful blood flow, making sure that you are energized and stay healthy. One study found that eating pomegranates on a regular basis helps men with erectile dysfunction, so go ahead and add it to your diet! Plus, there is nothing quite like eating these seeds off your lover's body.

Pumpkin Seeds

These little gems are rich in magnesium content – in fact, they are perhaps the richest in magnesium in most food categories. Magnesium, when taken in the right dosage, is brilliant for an active sex life – it increases the testosterone levels by making sure that more amount of testosterone enters your blood streams and keeps it flowing.

Drinks Champagne or red wine helps boost the sex drive. But too much alcohol is not recommended as it can affect your sex drive adversely.

Bananas

This fruit contains plenty of phosphorus and chelating minerals. This helps improve libido. In addition, it contains plenty of vitamins. So, if you have nothing else to try out, go for bananas to make your night wild.

Exercise daily

Wake up early in the morning. Use any mechanism possible but rise up and do some meditation. This makes your mind free from negative thoughts. First, the movement of your limbs and body will shake up your internal organs. It will revitalize them and improve the blood flow. You burn up the excess energy that would otherwise become fat. This makes you hungrier and your metabolism improves.

Plan your itinerary

It helps if you keep a watch over your daily schedule. If you set aside ten minutes for a walk, it makes you mentally prepared every day for the walk. In the same way, if you set aside thirty to forty minutes for lovemaking, it will help your mind to get attuned to the activity. After a few days, you can make adjustments to this item by adding time or adding the type of sexual intercourse you will be doing.

Chapter 13: The Intricacies of Pleasure and Orgasms

What is pleasure, in its simplest form?

It's the enjoyable feeling of satisfaction you receive when a desire is fulfilled.

When you've been craving a slice of pizza all day, and you get off work, head straight to Pizza Hut, wait patiently for your order to finish, and take that first cheesy, meaty, greasy, glorious bite, THAT feeling right there is pleasure.

Psychology describes pleasure in terms of positive feedback. We are motivated to seek out what gives us pleasure and recreate those instances that have given us pleasure in the past.

For our purposes, first we need to understand pleasure in its physical form (although, its mental form is just as important, and we will see how the two cooperate).

Physical pleasure stems from our central nervous system, the network of neurons that transmit information from all parts of our bodies to our brains.

Nerve endings near the surface of our skin receive these signals first. The density of these nerve endings differ in various parts of our body.

Can you guess where one of the highest concentrations might be?

If you guessed your genitals, you just won the $1 million prize. Well, maybe just a million orgasms (I'd rather have the latter).

According to Ian Kerner, Ph. D., sex counselor, and best-selling author of She Comes First: The Thinking Man's Guide to Pleasuring a Woman, the penis contains about 4,000 nerve endings while the clitoris contains about 8,000 (he doesn't note how many in the whole vagina/vulva, but there are more in the outer lips, inner lips, vaginal entrance, and inside the vagina).

That's A LOT. It's no wonder these areas are so sensitive.

You may be thinking, "Alright cool, I'll just focus on mine and my partner's genitals the whole time and we will have amazing orgasms. That's what I figured anyway."

It's not that simple, or that boring. Sexual pleasure is complex, but that is what makes it such an exciting journey to navigate.

I prefer to think less in terms of having sex with my partner's body, and more in terms of having sex with their brain and their mind as well.

I know that sounds strange, but it makes sense considering the brain is where all of our pleasure signals end up.

Breaking Down Orgasms

The road to orgasm is navigated in terms of phases, with mental and physical pleasure playing a part throughout.

Sex researchers, Masters and Johnson, identified four stages to what they call the "sexual response cycle." These stages are Excitement, Plateau, Orgasm, and Resolution.

The following derives from WebMD, sprinkled with my take on each phase.

Stage 1 – Excitement (time frame: A few minutes to several hours)

This is when your body and mind recognize that **sexual tension is present.**

There are palpable sexual overtones, like when you are dancing with someone at a club, or holding hands walking home together, or lying in bed kissing and rubbing each other.

At this point, muscle tension increases. Sometimes you are not consciously aware of it, but your stomach may have tightened or your leg muscles may have stiffened up.

Your heart rate increases and your breathing becomes deeper.

WebMD states that your skin may become flushed, as in reddish blotches around the chest and back. (I have read this before, but I have never seen or noticed it. I have felt my skin getting warmer, however.)

The nipples harden (woot woot!).

Here's the big one: Blood flow to the genitals increases. The penis becomes erect and the clitoris/inner lips swell. Vaginal lubrication also begins (the vulva, or outer area of the vagina including the lips, clitoris, and vaginal entrance, gets "wet").

Breasts gain in size and the internal vaginal walls start to swell. Testicles also swell, the scrotum tightens, and fluid may secrete from the penis.

Phew!

Now that we're all excited, let's move on to Stage 2.

Stage 2 – Plateau

The plateau is everything from initial stimulation to the moment just before release, or orgasm.

You can view this whole process as a constant buildup of sexual tension, through teasing, give and take, multitasking, and some of the other techniques we'll discuss later which make up the meat of this guide.

In this phase, all of the changes that started in the Excitement phase increase in intensity.

The vulva swells further as blood flow increases. The clitoris becomes more sensitive, and may retract under the clitoral hood if it is overstimulated.

The testicles withdraw into the scrotum, and the penis reaches its maximum erection.

Your breathing, heart rate, and blood pressure increase. (What's interesting to note is that this happens even if the person isn't doing any physical activity during sex. I find that to be strong biological evidence for this part of the response cycle).

Muscle spasms may start to occur in places like the feet, face, hands, and thighs. Muscle tension increases further as well.

Stage 3 – Orgasm

The Big O. The Grand Finale. The Whole Shebang. The Thing We All Live For.

Ooorrrgaasmm.

It's when all of that built up tension and desire is released in one (and sometimes multiple) wave of intense feeling and pleasure. Hormones and endorphins flood the brain in a way that can only be described as pure ecstasy.

It's. Awesome.

And it's awesome giving it to someone else as well, but we'll get to that later.

What happens when we have an orgasm?

Involuntary muscle contractions begin, sometimes quite violently. Heart rate, blood pressure, and breathing reach their peak of intensity.

Muscles in the vagina contract, and the uterus also begins to contract.

Muscles contract at the base of the penis stimulating the ejaculation of semen.

Neurohormones (oxytocin and prolactin) are released, which are largely attributed to our feelings of intense pleasure when we have an orgasm. Endorphins are also released, contributing to the same result.

A reddish flush may appear all over the body, especially in the face.

Stage 4 – Resolution

Resolution is the comedown after climax. It's when your body's responses return back to their pre-excitement phase – i.e. back to normal.

It's also when you get that "Ahhhhh..." feeling of relaxation. Your muscles feel like jello, they are just tired enough to be fatigued, and you may feel heightened intimacy with your partner.

The **refractory period** also kicks in at this point. This is the period between the most recent orgasm and when the individual is physically capable of having another one or continuing stimulation.

It's a period where the person needs to rest and recuperate before they can continue more sexual activity.

This period differs for everyone, and even on a circumstantial basis and/or with age, but it is commonly an extended period of time for partners who have a penis. Ever heard partners of those who have a penis complain that their partner falls asleep or can't continue after having an orgasm? The refractory period plays a part in this.

It's important to note that everyone goes through these phases differently and feels them to varying degrees. While there may be a general framework for how everyone progresses to orgasm, we all feel physical pleasure differently, just how people gain pleasure from other things differently, such as pizza.

(I personally don't gain any pleasure from mushrooms. Italian sausage on the other hand…..wait a second. I'll be right back).

That's why communication about what each other likes is so important. It's also why different partners require, and offer a chance at, unique ways to bring them to the highest heights of pleasure.

You also feel pleasure differently than any partners your current partner may have had, so don't forget to tell them what works best for you as well.

As you may have noticed, the physical responses described in the sexual response cycle are largely involuntary. But they are just that – responses to the stimulation of an external force, whether you are stimulating yourself or someone else is stimulating you, and vice versa.

While specific pleasure responses are far from universal, there are MANY aspects of sex that can be applied to any situation.

This book is largely based on the techniques people can use to confidently find the right combination of sexual vehicles that will lead to great sex.

Great sex with most, if not any partner.

On to the meat of this guide: The need-to-knows of foreplay, oral sex, anal sex, powerful sex positions, sex toys, and dirty talk.

This portion of the guide is quite detailed. If you start to feel overwhelmed, read through it slowly, note the important points, and refer to it later when your mind has given the information a chance to sink in.

Chapter 14: The Most Intimate Positions For Couple

When you search for sex positions on the internet, you will find that most sources list the same positions over and over again. While this isn't necessarily a bad thing, they typically don't tell you why they chose them.

For our purposes, I'm only going to include the best of the best that I've found. These are the positions that provide the most pleasure, the hottest sex, the deepest intimacy, and give you the best opportunities to multitask (which will be discussed in a later chapter).

I have broken them up into penetrative, non-penetrative, and oral sex positions. Penetrative includes any object, such as a penis, toy, or strap-on dildo, being used to enter your partner. Non-penetrative includes the rubbing together of genitals and mutual masturbation.

I'll be describing the positions in terms of how both partners should be situated and what benefits each position offers.

Good sex requires different positions. Great sex requires POWERFUL positions.

Let's break 'em down.

Powerful Penetrative Positions

#1 Missionary With Legs in the Air

Description-

- The penetrating partner is on top and the receiving partner is on bottom.

- Instead of regular missionary with the receiving partner's legs spread out on the bed, the receiving partner spreads their legs about two feet apart and lifts them up in the air towards the ceiling, keeping them in front of their partner. Their body becomes an L shape.

- The receiving partner rests the back of their legs against the chest and shoulders of their partner, typically with their knees bending over their partner's shoulders and their hamstrings on their partner's chest.

- The penetrating partner leans forward, with their head between their partner's legs, and put their hands on the bed next to their partner's head, with their arms straight. This should angle their partner's pelvis upwards.

- Finally, the penetrating partner enters.

Benefits-

- Great angle for stimulating the G-Spot, anus, and/or prostate.
- The pressure of the receiving partner's legs provides some relief for the penetrating partner's arms.
- The receiving partner is somewhat constrained, which can be a turn on for many people.

Variation-

- Instead of two legs towards the ceiling, the receiving partner only puts one of their legs up, providing a different angle of stimulation.

#2 Missionary While Grabbing the Butt

Description-

- Regular missionary position with the penetrating partner on top and receiving partner on bottom, except the penetrating partner lies completely on top, resting their weight on their partner.

- With their head to the side of their partner's head, possibly resting on the pillow, the penetrating partner reaches down with both hands and grabs hold of their partner's butt.

Benefits-

- Allows the penetrating partner to pull their partner in towards them and thrust at the same time.
- Creates more bodily contact, increasing intimacy.
- Better angle than regular missionary for stimulating the G-Spot, anus, and/or prostate.

#3 Receiving Partner Lying Sideways and Penetrating Partner On Top

Description-

- The receiving partner lies on their side with legs bent at a 90 degree angle.
- The penetrating partner enters from the top, so the front of the penetrating partner is facing the side of the receiving partner.

- The penetrating partner kneels within the 90 degree angle of their partner's legs, positioning their pelvis to enter their partner.
- The penetrating partner leans forward and places their hands, arms, or elbows on both sides of their partner to hold themselves up.

Benefits-

- Different angle of stimulation.
- Can still kiss each other, heightening intimacy.

Variation-

- The penetrating partner grabs their partner's top leg and puts it over the corresponding arm.
- This widens either the vagina or anus for easier entry, and creates a different dynamic of constraint.

#4 Legs in the Air on the Edge of the Bed

Description-

- Similar to #1. The receiving partner lies on their back, puts their legs **together** and raises them up to the ceiling so their body is

in an L shape. Except this time, they are on the edge of the bed with the penetrating partner standing up.

- The penetrating partner wraps or holds on to their partner's legs for thrusting leverage, and may have to bend their knees down a bit to enter their partner. However, this partner does not lean over yet, like in #1, but stays standing straight.

Benefits-

- The penetrating partner gets great leverage by holding onto or wrapping around their partner's legs.
- Another optimal angle for stimulating the G-Spot, anus, and/or prostate.

Variation-

- Can have legs spread open rather than together.
- Can do the same as #1, with legs spread, hamstrings against the chest, and penetrating partner leaning over their partner while holding themselves up.

#5 Doggy Style With Receiving Partner Curling Towards Other Partner

Description-

- Receiving partner goes on their hands and knees while the penetrating partner gets on their knees and enters from behind.

- Instead of being on their hands, the receiving partner then rests one shoulder on the bed and angles their head to the opposite side, angling their back downwards towards the bed. The receiving partner should be able to look back and see their partner.

- The receiving partner rests their arms on the bed towards their partner.

- The penetrating partner holds on to their partner's hips for thrusting leverage.

Benefits-

- Better angle for deeper penetration.

- Increased arousal by both partners being able to lock eyes with one another, and especially for the receiving partner who gets to see their partner entering them from behind.

- Penetrating partner can get good leverage by holding onto their partner's hips and waist.

Variation-

- The receiving partner bends their knees further and lowers their pelvis down closer to the bed. They then reach back with their hands and wrap their arms around their legs, curling themselves further into a ball.

#6 Doggy Style With Penetrating Partner Squatting Over

Description-

- The receiving partner is on their hands and knees in doggy style position.

- Instead of being on their knees as well, the penetrating partner stands with their feet on either side of their partner, squatting down until they are at the right height to enter. The receiving partner may need to angle their pelvis upwards to help with entry.

- If the penetrating partner is comfortable, they can thrust like this. Otherwise, if they need more balance they can place their hands on the back, shoulders, or hips of their partner while squatting.

Benefits-

- Allows for deeper penetration.
- This angle from behind is better for hitting the G-Spot, anus, and/or prostate.
- The penetrating partner can use gravity to help them thrust.

Variation-

- Similar to the previous position (#5 - Doggy Style With Receiving Partner Curling Towards Other Partner), the receiving partner can angle their back down towards the bed, reach their arms back towards their partner, and curl themselves into a ball. This allows for further comfort during deep penetration and a different angle of stimulation. It also increases intimacy by being able to see each other's faces.

#7 From Behind With Receiving Partner Laying On Stomach

Description-

- The receiving partner lies flat on their stomach with their legs out straight and close together.
- The penetrating partner straddles their partner, with their knees on either side, leans forward, and uses their hands and arms to hold them up while entering their partner.

Benefits-

- Makes the vagina/anus tighten for increased pleasure of both partners.
- A comfortable position for both partners.
- Allows for a lot of multitasking, including hair pulling, kissing and sucking the neck/back, and manual stimulation (hand) of the genitals of the receiving partner.

Variation-

- The penetrating partner lies fully on the receiving partner, without holding themselves up, increasing bodily contact and intimacy.

- The penetrating partner can also reach under and provide manual stimulation to their partner's genitals.

- Provides opportunity to kiss from behind.

#8 Lying Down Sideways Penetration From Behind

Description-

- The receiving partner lies on their side with knees bent at around and 90 degree angle.

- The penetrating partner lies on their side behind them, entering as they would in regular doggy style and using their partner's hip(s) as leverage.

Benefits-

- Hugely intimate position, as it resembles cuddling.

- Provides a lot of opportunity for multitasking, including hair pulling, kissing from behind, manual stimulation of the genitals, and constraint by pulling back and locking the receiving partner's arms.

Variation-

- The penetrating partner lifts up the top leg of the receiving partner, either holding it up or placing it on top of their own. This expands the vagina/anus allowing for more comfortable penetration.

#9 Receiving Partner On Top (with variations)

Description-

- The penetrating partner lies on their back with the receiving partner straddling them.
- The receiving partner sits on their partner as they enter them.
- The receiving partner moves their body in a way that stimulates both partners.

Benefits-

- The receiving partner gets to control rhythm and stimulation.
- The receiving partner gains a more dominant role and can exercise more control.
- The penetrating partner becomes the more submissive role.

- The receiving partner is able to move in a way that best stimulates them, and can control the depth of penetration.

- Provides opportunity for either partner to manually stimulate the receiving partner's genitals in addition to penetration.

Variations-

- Instead of straddling their partner on their knees, the receiving partner squats over, bending their knees far enough to have their partner enter them. They can place their hands on their partner's shoulders, chest, stomach, or the pillow/bed for added stability and control.

- The receiving partner sits with full penetration and rolls their hips back and forth as they straddle their partner.

- The receiving partner moves up and down, similar to the thrusting action of the penetrating partner.

- The receiving partner lies forward with their weight on the penetrating partner, and rolls their body back and forth or moves up and down. The penetrating partner (on bottom) can also place their hands on their partner's hips or butt to control the rhythm.

- The receiving partner arches backward, instead of forward, and reaches backward placing their hands on either their partner's legs or the bed for balance. The receiving partner then moves in a way that is great for stimulating the G-Spot, anus, and/or prostate.

- The receiving partner faces the opposite direction while straddling their partner, with their butt facing their partner. The receiving partner can put their hands on either the bed or their partner's legs for added balance and control.

- The receiving partner faces the opposite direction, like before, but on their hands and feet facing the ceiling (so their back is towards their partner and they are in a "spider crawl" position). They then lower their hips down enough for their partner to enter. The penetrating partner relieves some of their partner's muscular strain by supporting their hips or lower back with their hands. The penetrating partner then uses that leverage to thrust.

Powerful Non-Penetrative Positions (Wikipedia)

#1 Rubbing Together of the Genitals

Description/Variations-

- One partner positions themselves in between their partner's thighs and rubs their genitals or a similar object (such as a strap-on dildo) on their partner's genitals.

- In the case of two people with vaginas, both people face each other positioning their legs to make contact with each other's vulva in order to rub them together. Sometimes called scissoring.

- In the case of two people with penises, both people position themselves in order to rub their penises together. Sometimes called frot or frottage.

Benefits-

- Risk of unwanted pregnancy dramatically decreases.

- Provides pleasure and intimacy for those who are uncomfortable with penetrative sexual activity.

#2 Mutual Masturbation

Description-

- Both partners lie next to each other in a way that provides easy manual stimulation of each other's genitals.
- Can lie on their backs, on their sides facing each other, both partners facing the same way, or with one partner on their back and the other on their side facing their partner.

Benefits-

- Risk of unwanted pregnancy dramatically decreases.
- Provides pleasure and intimacy for those who are uncomfortable with penetrative sexual activity.

Powerful Oral Sex Positions

#1 68-ing (variation of 69)

Description-

- Similar to the popular "69" position, where one partner lies on their back and the other straddles their genitals over their partner's face, facing the opposite direction and allowing oral access to both partner's genitals (can also be done side-by-side).
- One partner provides oral stimulation to the partner that is lying down, while they orient their body to give their partner manual access to stimulate their genitals.

Benefits-

- Good for foreplay and warming up both partners.

#2 Fellatio Variations

Description-

- The giving partner (the one performing the oral sex) lies on their back with their head hanging off the bed. The receiving partner (the one receiving the oral sex) enters their mouth while standing off the bed, allowing for thrusting. Receiving partner can also reach over and stimulate their partner's genitals at the same time. Can also be done with the giving partner lying on their stomach.

- The receiving partner (receiving oral sex) lies on their back with their legs hanging off the edge of the bed. The giving partner kneels off the bed and provides oral.

#3 Cunnilingus Variations

Description-

- The receiving partner lies on their back with a pillow (or multiple) under their butt in order to lift up their pelvis. The giving partner positions their head in between the thighs of the receiving partner.

- The receiving partner lies on their back with their legs hanging off the edge of the bed. The giving partner kneels off the bed and provides oral. The giving partner can also place the receiving partner's legs over their own shoulders.

Michael's Powerful Position

#1 Gravity

Description-

- I have never seen this position anywhere else, so as far as I'm concerned, I invented it. It's a penetrative position.

- The receiving partner is off the bed and places their shoulder blades on the ground (they are going to be practically upside down) with their back resting against the side of the bed. You may want to place a pillow underneath their head and shoulder blades.

- The receiving partner's legs are spread apart and in the air reaching towards the ceiling.

- The penetrating partner extends their legs on the bed, with their upper body hanging off the bed being supported in a horizontal manner by their hands and arms. They are now in a position to enter.

- The penetrating partner uses gravity to thrust every time they move their hips up towards the ceiling and back down.

Benefits-

- It's awesome.

Note that any of these positions can be adapted to use sex toys as well. And when attempting a new position, make sure you're taking the necessary safety precautions not to injure yourself or your partner. Some positions are acrobatic endeavors.

When you first start learning new positions, I suggest taking them one by one instead of trying to go through all of them in a single session. It can be a little stressful trying to remember ten new positions you learned that day. Focus on one at a time and you will memorize each as they become a part of your sexual arsenal.

And don't forget to have fun. Trying new positions is a great activity to share with your partner or partners. Talk about them, play around with what works and what doesn't, and find the top rotation of positions you can stick to that provide the most fun and pleasure.

Can you guess what's next?

Toys!

And no, not the Legos you used to play with. Although, I'm sure you could make something useful out of them for the bedroom.

Conclusion

If I had to pick a few main points that I think you should take away from reading this book, they would be as follows:

-Women want you to take your time and warm them up as much as possible. Do not rush sex with a woman. Quickies are fine but unless she is wet and ready the experience will not be optimal.

-Men and women both love spontaneity. Do not get into a bland routine. Try new things, especially by having sex in different and exciting places. Give your man a blowjob when he least expects it and he is sure to return the favor.

-Men are very visual, they like seeing your whole body and they love it when you are vocal during sex. Tell your man to "do you harder," to "spank you," to make you cum hard." Moan and yell your man's name and they are sure to repay you with intense sex. While giving your man head try to let him see your entire body. Suck him at an angle and let him see your bum and breasts. Do 69 with your man and allow your vagina to be directly in his face.

-Make sex a learning experience. Many couples feel that when they begin having sex, they enter a different realm. Do not allow yourself to get into this mindset. By making sex a different interaction you make it more difficult to communicate normally. Don't be afraid to laugh and joke during sex from time to time, this will lighten the mood and make it easier to vocalize exactly what you want in bed. Make time during sex to have a quick discussion on what you both want, don't want and what you might like to try.

-Watch each other masturbate. This can be an extremely helpful practice as it gives you visual information on what your partner truly likes. Sometimes it's difficult for a person to put into words how they want to be pleasured. By showing your partner what you like you leave little room for misinterpretation.

-Try anything once as long as it's not painful or potentially harmful. You should always let your partner know that he/she will not be judged for suggesting something new and taboo. Maybe you're a woman and you want to have sex with your man in front of another person, who videotapes the event, or maybe you're a man and you really want to have anal sex with your woman and you would also like her to give you a prostate massage. No matter what the suggestion is, make sure your partner knows that it's perfectly okay to suggest new sexual ideas. It's also perfectly okay to say no to ideas but I think having the rule of trying anything once (as long as it isn't painful or if it REALLY makes you uncomfortable) is a good idea. By trying anything once your partner will respect you. Let's say you try anal sex at your partner's request and you don't enjoy it. Your partner should not ask you to try it again since you have already tried and disliked it. You must respect your partner's likes and dislikes and keep an open, nonjudgmental environment in the bedroom at all times.

Sex is an important part of life and crucial for being in a fulfilling relationship. Whether you have a great sex life and just want to keep experimenting, or you're just starting to explore what makes you and your partner feel good, I hope this book has been a useful resource for you. Don't forget that this book is only a start. By opening up communication with your partner about sex, you can both continue to explore and grow sexually, figuring out how to have the most satisfying sexual relationship possible. Sex is for everyone, from flexible yogis to couch potatoes, so wink at your partner, shimmy out of your clothes, and start having fun!

www.ingramcontent.com/pod-product-compliance
Lightning Source LLC
Chambersburg PA
CBHW070901080526
44589CB00013B/1156